What Weight

J.M. Clark

iUniverse, Inc.
New York   Bloomington

What Weight

The information, ideas, and suggestions in this book are not intended as a substitute for professional medical advice. Before following any suggestions contained in this book, you should consult your personal physician. Neither the author nor the publisher shall be liable or responsible for any loss or damage allegedly arising as a consequence of your use or application of any information or suggestions in this book.

iUniverse books may be ordered through booksellers or by contacting:

iUniverse
1663 Liberty Drive
Bloomington, IN 47403
www.iuniverse.com
1-800-Authors (1-800-288-4677)

Because of the dynamic nature of the Internet, any Web addresses or links contained in this book may have changed since publication and may no longer be valid. The views expressed in this work are solely those of the author and do not necessarily reflect the views of the publisher, and the publisher hereby disclaims any responsibility for them.

ISBN: 978-1-4502-3585-3 (sc)
ISBN: 978-1-4502-3590-7 (ebook)

Printed in the United States of America

iUniverse rev. date: 5/26/2010

Reality Hurts

When it came to a beginning for my book, I thought I would tell the readers about when I had my first stroke. I mention at this time, that nothing that I tell the readers in this book, has been easy for me to write, even after three years, and my losing over 370 pounds. It took much determination, and my faith in believing, that others are out there in need of this book, supplying me with the courage, I needed to enable me to write it. When it came to me having a stroke, nothing came easy; not when I was going through it, or even now that I have lived through it. Fear is dangerous. I will talk more on fear later, but each day I live with the fear or the nightmare, that I could no matter what I have done to improve my health, still have another stroke. For having that stroke for me; was the beginning of a real nightmare, and started the cycle of change in my life. At my first stroke, I was 43 years old, weighed in at over four hundred pounds (my actual weight at this time was 575.9 pounds. (Why do women like to hide their true weight?), and was suffering from arthritis, COPD, pinch nerves, and bone deterioration.

I was happy (with many days of deep depression, which I covered by overeating and drinking); I thought nothing of my weight at this time; for I considered it to be normal for me (I had been living with this weight for years). As most readers can relate, I had taken my weight problem and made it normal. Everyone around me kept trying to inspire me to lose weight, but it was useless talk, for I had tuned them out; I felt I was normal and often would say "God made me this way, so I don't have a problem with it!" The truth of the matter was God hadn't made me this way; I had become overweight over the years as I overate, and overstuffed myself into believing, that I *needed the food to survive.* Yes, I convinced myself that I needed the food I was eating, because I was a big woman; and it took more to satisfy my hunger. Have you too often thought this? Have you been giving yourself excuses? The night before my stroke, I had given a party for my daughter, and my grandchildren, at my apartment. I love cooking, and was running my own catering business on the side; so it didn't take much to encourage me to get into the kitchen. I remember my grandchildren and I had stayed up until three in the morning; we were lost laughing, and watching scary movies, and eating popcorn, which I had doctored up with chili spices and hot butter. Popcorn would not be complete without hot chocolate, with extra marshmallows and whipped cream. I had made homemade pizza dough, and had topped the two pizzas, with nearly everything I had in the fridge. We were so full, that we all were lying around on the floor, nursing our hurting stomachs and waiting for the antacid to work. I thought I would burst; I took my bicarbonate, and waited patiently for the blurb of relief. Only a few hours went by, and I was up preparing for breakfast that morning. I made pancakes, with extra butter and warmed syrup, sausages, bacon and orange juice (which I would mix with pineapple juice). I must have eaten nine pancakes and five sausages that morning. To make matters even worst I put a shot of Vodka (the hair of the dog from the night before) and mixed it in my juice. I remember drinking two large eight ounce glasses of that juice that morning.

I want the reader to understand just how much I was eating and how I accepted it as normal. This was very embarrassing for me to write about; mainly because it meant the reader would know how big of a pig I was. I would have left it out all together, but the truth of the matter is that I needed to tell the truth. How many readers face the same dilemma I went through thinking it was normal? Have you too been hiding behind that extra pancake and sausage? I remember letting my grandchildren out the door that morning, and turning and looking at the mess in the kitchen. (At that time I lived in a one bedroom apartment and the kitchen was the first thing you saw when you walked through the door.) I turned to go clean up the mess on the table, and the floor, which the four year old had left behind. I suddenly had the sharpest pain in my chest; I remember grabbing at my chest because the pain was so sharp. I also seem to remember feeling something shooting down my arm; it felt like my arm was coming off my body. I remember the pain in my chest, was suddenly so great, I went crashing to the floor. I was a woman, weighing over four hundred pounds, so when I hit that floor; I hit hard. (I had a beautiful blue vase that sat on a cocktail stand, and when I fell to the floor the vibrations knocked the vase to the floor, smashing it into a million pieces.) I can't tell you how long I was out or unconscious, but I am grateful that I woke up. I was lying on the floor, and I had this horrible pain and stiffness all over my body. I tried to stand but I couldn't move, I tried to holler for help, but my mouth was not opening. I looked all around for something which could get someone's attention. But even when I found something I couldn't move, and found myself for the first time in my life, feeling a fear, that I had never encountered before. I knew I was unable to help myself, and I was terrified. There are no words to explain how I felt or how hard it was for me to move forward. I was a woman who was pass fear I was terrified. The only thing, that seems to be keeping me going, was the fact I could hear this pastor, on the radio saying; that a change was coming, and warning the listener not to give up. "Keep trying to reach your goal…" He went on and on in this high pitch, country dragging, squeaky, and rather annoying voice. I remember thinking I wish he would shut up, yet as I laid there on the floor; I began to wish he could reach through that radio, and help me up off the floor. I lay on that floor for over twelve hours. I spent that Sunday listening to minister after minister, preach on hope and not giving up on life. I begged God to help me and promised I would try to do better with my life "Mind you I usually would promise God I would do better, and I had good intentions, but once feeling better I would soon forget my promise." There was no one to come to help me for I was such a private person and kept to myself (mainly because of my size). I was always the life of the party, but the truth of the matter was, I was really a rather lonely woman. I spent most of my time alone. I waited hour after hour, for someone to pass by my window, or knock on my door but no one came. I laid there struggling to get up and feeling at a lost that I was unable to move. I prayed that I would be able to holler at that time, if someone came and let them know I was inside in trouble. Then the nightmare of me being stuck on the floor would be over. During the time I was waiting I was trying to get off the floor, but the only thing I was succeeding at doing was giving my body a severe carpet burn. I had used the restroom and I had no control over my bladder or bowel movements.

I was a vain woman and I dreaded anyone finding me in this condition. I when needing the most help, *was still to vain*. I can only tell you that after I humbled myself, accepted the fact that I needed to get help in learning how to control my eating; suddenly I began to feel movement in my legs and arms. I began to drag myself over to the sofa. (The sofa was only about three feet away, yet it took me hours to reach it; and the pain I was feeling from the carpet burns, were indescribable). Up until this point in my life, I must admit that I believed in God, but I felt that I was in control of my life; and that I was happy, so I didn't take kindly, or respect anyone trying to influence me on the matter. I began to think about all of the things I was doing wrong, along with those things that I knew I shouldn't be doing, or could be doing much better. I really put my life on the fore front, and as I did I began to feel a change in my heart. I knew I had changed, I knew I believed I could get up off of the floor. Lying on that floor had humbled and made me realize that I not only needed help, that I wanted the help. I wanted to get better; I wanted to lose the weight.

I felt I was in control, but as I lay there on that floor, I saw myself, and I knew I had to make a change. I still could not get up off that floor, and I still could not talk. (Over four more hours passed) I wondered when someone would come to my house again. Because of the weight, I wasn't much on having company (except for family), or going to many places (no one wants to ride an overweight person in their car); so I knew I was in for a long wait, especially when it came to someone knocking on my door. By this time, I was soaked with urine, and I was soaking wet with perspiration from trying to get off the floor. My pride, had long since flew out of the window, and I was pass feeling self pity for myself. I was mad. I had everything to live for, and I was not going to let this problem conquer me. I felt I had to change in order to win. I am not a good loser. I believe that everyone; has something they are good at in their life. My pride, had been a problem for years; and I now had to face myself. I didn't like what I saw. I reviewed my life while lying on that floor, and what I saw, and now understand was hard to accept for my own good. For years I had hidden myself behind the food, I knew I could no longer hide; I had to step up and face the truth. It was Sunday evening, around ten o'clock, when my boyfriend, stumbled into my apartment in an alcoholic state.

This was not uncommon for him on a weekend; he usually would really tie one on. Who could blame him? He had been toting a four hundred pound woman around all week, on top of trying to hold down a job. He usually would treat me like a queen, except when he had too much to drink, then his true feelings would surface. Thus, what led to what happen that evening when he came into the apartment, and saw me on the floor. He looked at me lying on the floor, told me to get up, and get cleaned up, that I smelled bad. (Here I had waited for hours for help and this was what I received) I wanted to hit him on the head with the flower pot, but I couldn't reach him, or even speak yet. Just then on the radio, a minister yelled out, "Reach for God, he is the only one who will help you…Reach up and he will lift you up. Reach higher for he is waiting to help you…Believe in the impossible… REACH!" I can't explain it, I knew suddenly I could get up, and that I was going to do what the man had said. I *now believed in the impossible!*

I grabbed hold of the cushion on that sofa, and I began to pull myself off the floor. It took about an hour for me to succeed, and I knew I was going to have to throw the sofa out; because it was now ruined from the urine and bowel soiled clothing. I laid there for about another hour, and during that time I began to feel my legs. Tears of joy ran from my eyes, as my legs and arms began to get some feeling. (Two hours later) I soon had control; I thought as I made it to the bathroom, and into the tub. (I must have filled that tub with every smelling salt, bubble bath, scented oil that I had). Now, while I was in the tub, trying to clean up the horrible smell, which was coming from my body (even after the clothes were removed the smell seemed to linger on). I suddenly began having the worst spasms in my legs and feet. The pain was crippling, and all I could think to do was run the water, as hot as I could take it, in the hope that the hot water would help give me some relief. (I to this day, still suffer from these acute spasms and I have lost over 370 pounds, the doctors have been unable to tell me why I have these spasms, and I tire from all of the pain pills, and medicine they have no ideal will work, but enjoy testing it out on you anyway.) I want to say that I do believe in medicine, and even now doctors; but in all sincerity I still believe that they test too many drugs out on us, before they know all the good or bad of the drug. When it comes to overweight and excessively obese people, we stand as the world's prime targets.

It took me over two hours to bathe, and then to be able to pull my big behind out of the tub (I say this in humor now, though at the time it was not at all funny), and dry off. Thank God, I had a chair in the bathroom, and was able to sit on it, and successfully dry my body off (It took me nearly an hour to dry off). During all of this time, I had continuously, tried to call out to my boyfriend numerous times, in order to get his help; which I had long since conceded I needed. I was unable to do so, I still had no voice, and I was scared. Would I ever talk again? Or, my God, was this to be my fate?

When I came into my bedroom, I found my boyfriend passed out on the bed. I looked at him and then lay down, and thanked God for helping me. I laid there in my bed, smelling the liquor from my friend's mouth, as he loudly snored (For the first time in months, I was happy to hear and smell the horrible scent that morning.) As I drifted to sleep, I wondered would my voice be back when I awoke? I had no idea what the morning would bring, but I knew I would have to deal with it.

I woke twelve hours later, my body still sore, and my voice had not come back yet. I was embarrassed. I didn't want to tell anyone what had happened to me, but there were problems to still deal with. It took several hours into the day (much praying and pleading for help to God or any presence which could help me), before my voice did begin to come back. I was having trouble speaking, and something had happen to the sound of my voice. I had a very heavy accent, which confused me, for I didn't recognize my own voice. (I kept looking around for the person who was talking) I didn't understand where the sound was coming from, and more than that; I wasn't able to get control of the pain, which came from my throat. Even with all this vanity was still with me. I just didn't want people to know I had been trapped on the floor. I was suffering, inside as well as out. I began to feel a numbing in my arms again, and I had carpet burns all over my body. (My daughter feared I would get an infection from all of the wounds) It didn't make sense for me to not go to the doctor, wasn't it important to see what had happen to me? I had a bigger problem, when it came to doctors, because they had treated me so badly because of my size, that I didn't trust them or their judgment. (I can't tell you how many times I had a doctor insult me and call me fat, and tell me that I would never lose weight, because I didn't want to give up the food.)

I knew I needed to see a doctor (after three days and not much change, the pain now almost too hard to endure); I got dressed, and went to see the doctor. My regular doctor was out for the day and I knew that I would not do this again if I went home unseen). I agreed to see another doctor on staff, I told him what had happen, as best as I could remember; and he ran a few tests, then told me the results showed I had suffered a mild stroke. He went on to tell me that because of my weight, he didn't think I was going to make the year out without a change. I was told I needed to start a diet, and stick to it. He had no feelings at all he was so unemotional and seem to be looking right through me, I knew he didn't care that he was just doing his regular speech to an overweight person. He dismissed me like I was a fly being swatted with a fly swatter. I knew he was right, but I still wasn't ready to change. The most aggregating thing in my life has been going to the doctor; then having him tell me that I was too fat. I think doctors need to practice how to tell someone who is overweight, in a better way that they need help so as not to insult them. ***Insulting me will not make me listen and lose anything!*** *Overeating is a disease, and America needs to wake up and realize the seriousness of the matter.*

I left the doctor's office, and went next door to the Burger King, and brought a whopper with cheese, fries and coke and ate then went home. I got home and started dinner fried chicken, scallop potatoes and greens. You see even though I knew I had suffered a stroke, I was alright now. So the doctor told me I was placing my heart into danger, but he also insulted me, so I don't think I cared, or wanted to listen to him or anything he had to say. There were all kinds of signs that something was wrong, but I kept going on as though nothing was the matter with me. Two months went by, before I had another attack, and this time it brought me not only to my knees, it brought me to my senses. Once again I was stuck unable to help myself only this time I went to a hospital. I walked out of that hospital not only scared, but fully aware, that it was by the grace of God, that I know existed. I didn't know where to begin, but I knew I had to get the weight off; especially if I wanted to go on living. I tried diet after diet, and nothing was working. I was gaining weight. I was cooking healthy, so why wasn't I losing weight?

Before anyone can lose weight; you must first be in touch with the reality of what it takes to lose weight. The first and foremost important thing, is accepting you have to change your life. You have to begin again, a fresh new start; one that you yourself will guide and direct. Before you can do that, you must first learn what steps are necessary, to changing into a healthier lifestyle. Yes, as with anything else, beginning a change in your life is a step, and accepting you must change, in order to win the battle of being unhealthy.

I can't stress how serious it is to accept the fact you must make changes to your life, and those changes are important to your success. I, for years thought I could lose the weight, but I wouldn't give up the foods I liked. I am a woman of small means, and a wonderful meal is a luxury, I can afford to enjoy. I love to cook, and even worse, is the fact I am a taster. By the time the meal is finished, I have already tasted enough food, that none is needed when it comes to fixing my plate. It took me months to begin to find my way through the maze, and learn some tips, which could help not only me, but everyone who finds themselves in my position. Change isn't easy, but it is something that all of us can do, with a little help. To change your eating habits, one first must learn what they were doing wrong, so they can put a new plan into motion.

You can't change, until you know what you have to change. For most of us, it will take time to adjust to the steps, which will lead us to a new life. I brought a ton of books on weight loss, and read every one, but it didn't help much. I was learning some new tips, but I still wasn't losing weight. I couldn't understand since I was cooking healthy, why wasn't the weight beginning to come off? One reason was that I was still overeating, secondly, I still wasn't burning enough calories, to jump start my body into losing. The first thing I did, and that I suggest others try, is carrying around measuring cups. I had to learn what the proper amount of food was. I was so use to overeating that I found it hard to dial down to the proper amount. We live in a world where overeating is normal, and so it is hard for one to learn control, and stick to it. The measuring cups help do just that. They teach you portion control and more than that they help you learn what is normal.

I had been eating for three people instead of one, by the time I learned how much I was overeating; and what a real portion was, I began to see a light at the end of the tunnel. It took me three months of practicing with the measuring cups, before I could actually put the right amount on my plate without over doing it. Once I had learned the right portion, I then began to research the art of burning calories. I use to eat and then sit back and watch television, and I basically still do that; now I have learned a ton of exercises, that I do while sitting in front of the television. I burn calories sitting down. It took only three weeks of exercise, along with correct portion control and I saw the pounds begin to come off. Why did I tell you all this? *I wanted you to realize that problems come in all different ways and stages in our life. It is how we react to those problems, which create the problems or solve the problems we encounter. No one can be free of problems or circumstances in life, but we can learn to handle those circumstances, and advance forward with hope on winning the battle.*

Humor, is something all of us live with and need, but for those losing weight, humor is the key to success. When you can laugh at your problems, and see the humor in what you are attempting; you will see that losing weight is only changing your habits. Change is easy, when you can laugh your way through it, to your goal of success. I hope as you read on, you will begin to laugh along with me, at the problems that I encountered as I learned what it takes to take the weight off. Key one, and the most important key, is to learn to laugh at yourself, and accept as a child; that you must start over in order to succeed. *Yes, you could order some other control food program; but times are tough and the money is short. Wouldn't you rather learn to eat your way thin, and know that you will not gain the weight back, because you properly took the weight off yourself?* **Only you can take this first step, and it's the one that is the most important. You can accept the truth a little easier if you understand the problem. Consider taking the first step now!**

Secondly you must be straight with yourself. When it comes to weight loss, honesty with oneself is important. When you monitor yourself you help yourself to get control. A good way to get control of a situation is to keep a journal. It helps to write down how you are feeling about things, as you progress through reaching your goal. If you are seeking around and hiding food, you are only hurting yourself. You have to make a commitment to yourself that you will follow though to the end. You can soon understand where you need help, as your record your ups and downs. Everyone has days when they are just not with the program, but when you know how to control the food you are eating, and understand why you swayed, control becomes easier and your goal, becomes acceptable and obtainable.

Thirdly, stay away from the scale. Sure you need to know your beginning weight, but after that you should keep off the scale. Weighing in once a month is more than enough, you need to be inspired, and getting on the scale everyday will only stress you out. I believe that the stress that comes from looking down at your weight, day after day, will only defeat you. I weighed myself once a month and it was more than enough.

Fourth, you need to drink water, it not only helps with keeping you full, and it also aids in digestion, and keeps your body nourished and resilient. Here are some tips that might help if you are not a big water drinker:

Try adding some lemon, mint leaves, cucumber slices, chunks of fruit or you can use frozen grapes. These may seem like simple things but they help keep you focus and on point. Water is important but remember, that water also is taken into the body through fruits, and vegetables too. I wasn't much of a water drinker, so I like putting frozen grapes and slices of peaches or pineapple in my water. I let it sit in the fridge for about an hour, and then I kick back and enjoy the flavor. Sometimes I make lemonade out of real lemons, cayenne pepper and sugar substitute. The pepper believe it or not helps cut the appetite, I found I like ¼ teaspoon to a quart of water. I like my water over ice and very, very cold.

Fifth, be willing to make an attitude adjustment. You decided to lose the weight, now make the decision to change your way of thinking, by learning more about healthy living. Don't overdue your weight goal. I started small and increased my lost by a pound or two. I didn't want to get upset if I didn't lose anything. I just wanted to make sure I could make it happen, and you will too, once you start putting things into practice, you will welcome the new attitude. I found that I was nicer to people, I wasn't so sharp with them anymore. I worked on an overall makeover. I wanted to look good on the outside as well as in the inside. You have to really be willing to make a change inside and out, in order to get control of your inner being. The heart and the mind rule the stomach, not the other way around.

Sixth, learn to move around. Don't just sit there waiting for the weight to drop off. Sure you might lose a pound or two, but if you really want to see the pounds drop off, Try exercising more often. You can learn low impact exercises and do them in front of the television, sitting at the computer, sitting around the community room, exercise can be fun. You should take time to learn to work out to music; it helps you to keep a beat, and simply makes you feel good. Music is the key to a powerful workout. I have lost over 370 pounds and because the weight came off so quickly after I had Bariatric surgery, I was left with a lot of excess skin. The state of Michigan was willing to save my life, but not get rid my body of the excess skin, if I had known that I was going to look like a prune by the thighs, I would have started an exercise program much sooner than when I did. I have been learning to tone and stretch the muscle tissue. My skin really does look a lot better, but I have a long way to go. I don't think I will ever get rid of all of the skin, but I am attempting it. One of the problems of having bariatric surgery is if you can't afford to have your skin sculptured, you are left with an unsightly mess, unless you have been on a strict exercise program. I was so heavy that it was hard for me to get around at first. Once the weight started coming off I started walking around my neighborhood park. I could barely get around the park, which isn't even a mile. It would take me nearly two hours to walk once around it. I wish I had started weight training and toning sooner. Exercise and food go together; if you eat you need to be able to work it off. When you don't exercise you only add to the problem, and the only one who gets hurt in the end is you. It doesn't matter if you can't do a lot at first, what is important is that you do the exercises regularly.

Seventh, Take time to make each meal a chef's delight. If it looks good, then you can be assured of one thing, you will stick to the program and stay in control. Bland food will only make you want to go out and buy something with taste. Learn to use your spices and herbs to flavor your food. Keep in mind that black pepper is good for digestion, and that garlic helps in lowering your blood pressure. Take time to learn what each spice does in a dish and then try it out. Some you will like and others you won't, but just keep trying until you find the spices that you do like. I wasn't much for tarragon, but I love basil and thyme. I put basil in my tea, in my water, in my sauces; and to cut my appetite when I feel a little too hungry, in between meals I chew on some fresh basil leaves. I fix myself all kinds of relish trays and fruit trays and sit them in the fridge. When I get a little hunger attack, I just go to the fridge and nibble on something from my tray.

Eighth, learn to roll with your mistakes. So you have a little set back, so what! Learn to accept that losing weight takes persistence, patience, and time in order for you to change. Don't waste your time feeling guilty about a mistake, or a setback. Just start over again, adjust your meals accordingly, and continue on. Learn from your mistakes; reflect on your day with hope and courage for a new one. Your mind will play a huge part in your accepting the new. Control is easy once you know the simple basics, which helps the mind say yes to eating habits. You first must accept that you can concur this matter of learning control the change.

These steps are not full proof, but I stuck to them and found them to work. I pass them on to you in the hope that you will find one or two acceptable for you. No I am no doctor, so I expect you to check what I am saying out with your doctor. I have never showed or taught anyone anything that I haven't learned and done for myself first. I made many mistakes and had many setbacks. I gained twenty pounds back, during rough time in my life. I just started over again, and I have never held one of my mistakes over my head. I figured if I approached things like a child, and forgave myself with the childlike innocence children have, that I could do it. No diet is perfect, but what I have learned is that if you don't learn it for yourself; that you will find yourself gaining the weight back. One of the problems I have found with the paid food programs, were the fact when you can't pay for the program's food, they cut you off cold. Now if you have been simply eating the food they sent, you will find yourself suddenly at a lost when you go to the grocery store. Many of the people I talked to, who gained their weight back, said it was because they didn't know anything about cooking the food, and they were surprised at the price of the grocery bill, when they tried to prepare the meals themselves. There is an old saying that I teach at my club meetings, "Once learned, never forgotten. If you never learn anything, for sure you won't have anything to remember."

A Closer Look at What Weight Is in Relationship to Your Life

One of the most amazing things in life is the knowledge that we live in a world of complete selfishness, and it doesn't appear to be getting any better. I keep asking myself, how can I help others realize that dieting is easy? That for the most part, it's just learning how to eat correctly, that we lack an understanding of. Most of us, need to learn the basics, but for half, the chance of that happening is slim. We have such high levels of pride and such high vanity issues, that we won't admit we need help. From the time we are children, we are taught to eat what is sat before us. You knew better than to question your mother, about it being something you didn't want. Our parents, and most of society, seems stuck on learning the food groups, but not the correct food amounts which will keep you satisfied, and not put weight on you. You would think parents would want to teach their children how to properly eat the right portion of food. (Especially, when you look at all of the overweight children, and teenagers in society today. McDonalds, and all the other fast food companies, though they are trying hard to improve on the mess they created; have only added to the problem. They are still overfilling the plates, and mixing the wrong things together and calling it healthy.) Do you truly know what Healthy living is all about?

Look at the amount of food we are given at restaurants, and eateries. The enormous amount of food, they pile on the plate, and set before us as a normal portion. Have you ever questioned having too much food on your plate? (I know I never questions the over amount, but just let it be short, and all hell would break out). Just as bad, is the fact, that most of us have been program to eat all of the food, which is set in front of us. I can still remember my mother saying "eat everything that is on your plate. " Can't you remember your parents doing the same? Can't you remember your mother giving you the eye of death, when you did mention something? How many times did you take time to hide the food which you didn't like? Strange, how as children we know when to say we are full, yet as adults something happens to that knowledge; and we are lost spending money to learn how to do just that.

My mother would often remind us that there were children in the world going hungry. Now I know that there is a problem in the world with people eating too much, and that there is also a problem with people eating too little. Regardless to whatever one may say; this problem has existed since the beginning of time. There have been homeless people, children needing a home, and someone to love them, abuse, hatred and the list goes on and on, since time, as we know it began. People have been making the same mistakes, over and over again, for centuries. The way we address the problem changes, but everything else remains the same. The possibility of anyone solving the world's problems seems far from one's mind, or reality. All of the above statements; are meant to trigger some inner thoughts and emotions. I want you to consider what I am saying, and whether you yourself might have the same problems, when it comes to food and your relationship with food. Do you find yourself overeating and not knowing when to stop? Are you scared that you will go hungry? Have something happen in your life, which has been so traumatic that you find yourself eating; in order to simply deal with the problem? Are you one who munches? Under pressure do you turn to putting food into your mouth?

I am not going to be able to change the world; but I can help correct the problems place there by man; in teaching the wrong principles, when it comes to food and how we should consume it. Sure, we should teach the basic food groups, but along with that, we should teach what the proper amount of food we should consume is. For instance, we should teach the importance of milk, or consuming calcium; but we should also teach that it is not necessary to consume eight ounces when all you need is four. (There are many ways to consume calcium and get our daily intake. Vegetables and fruits are high in calcium.) I agree with the facts, that children need more milk or calcium, because of their growing bones. (But we are only children for a short time).Or how about toast, sure we need starch in our lives; but we don't need two slices of bread in the morning, we could live with just having one slice with our meal. I find that we eat double or triple what we should be consuming. When the proper amount is set in front of us we have already program ourselves into believing that it is not enough; and that we must consume more in order to be satisfied.

How many times have you ordered something at a restaurant, and then when it arrives, you question why there is so little on your plate? I remember sending my plate back once, and demanding the manager to put more food on it. I couldn't believe he tried to cheat me, and I was furious. When the manager tried to explain that I had the correct portion on my plate; I became enraged. How dare he try to starve me? Didn't he know I was hungry and needed to eat? What was even more amazing was that I couldn't eat all of the food that was on my plate. The portion they had given me had been enough; only I had been brained washed, into believing that I had to have more in order to get full. Do you know when your body has had enough? Or are you one of those people who eats until you feel like you're going to bust? I think for the most part we all over eat, and that unless you are made aware of the fact you are overeating; that you would never question it. How many times have you sat back and unbuckled your belt, in order to just get more food into you? "Oh just one more bite", we say as we try to stuff that fork full of food into our mouths. Come on, can that one bite really fills you? What makes us think that we can be full with just one more bite?

One of the things that I teach in my health club (WALKRFREE ROTATING HEALTH CLUB, started in 2006 to help seniors and the handicap, who needed help in portion control and more information on healthy living.)I review the importance of knowing how much food is needed in order for the body to properly maintain itself. I encourage each person to go and pick up a measuring cup set, and teach them to look at what 1(one) cup of food, looks like on their plate. I know that many of us don't want to go inside of a restaurant, and pull out that cup, and start measuring. So the next best thing is to learn, what one cup of food really looks like. Memorize it, and then start putting that method of control into our lives. You have to start somewhere, so why not begin with learning the correct portions you should be eating? In the privacy of your home, you can teach yourself portion control, without anyone's interference. You can really pay attention to what a portion control plate of food looks like. This will help you when you go out to restaurants and eateries, not to overeat, but to consume what is only necessary for you to live on.

I use to get mad, when someone would say you have too much on your plate. Now, I say thank you, and I readjust my way of thinking. This is what is important, not how much, but how I react to what is in front of me, whether I am at home, or in another surrounding. So in this chapter, we will deal with portion control; mainly because **portion** control is what will help you get *control.* You already know all the different foods you like and dislike what I will teach you are how to eat them without hurting yourself. So let's get ready to start learning how much food is legal, and putting that knowledge into our brains. For some, reading this once will be enough*; for others you will have to read it two or three times in order to* **get it.** So what, it doesn't matter how many times you have to study it; the point is that you will study, and learn what is important. ***The very first thing is to stop saying I am on a diet, but to say I am learning how*** *to eat* **correctly**. Diet, is simply a four letter word that man has put too much emphasis on. ***Learning to eat* is *fun,*** and I am going to have you laughing your way into a smaller size. If you think you can't laugh your way into knowledge, then keep reading, and you will soon see that you can, and will do so.

One of my most embarrassing moments with my measuring cups was when I first started using them. I was invited out to dinner; it was a big function down at the church. I reached into my purse and pulled out the measuring cup and started filling it with the food from off my plate. One of the senior's, noticing me walked over and told me that I didn't have to bring cups from home, that they had plenty of food and cleaned plates. I was embarrassed because up until then when he mentioned it, no one had even noticed what I was doing. You see, I was embarrassed because I needed help. I couldn't recognize what a cup of food looked like, and hadn't considered, what I would do, if someone asked what I was doing. Portion control is something which you will find at first is hard to accept, but don't let that, or your embarrassing moments stop you. You must learn to recognize what a control amount of food looks like, and more than that you must be satisfied with it. I hope you will go out and buy your measuring cups today. Today is your first days of discovery…make it one you will be proud of.

The measuring cups are not the only tools; we have to learn with, we have our hands. Look at the palm of your hand; take a good look at that palm. Your palm is the correct size of your portion of meat. It should be able to fix in the palm of your hand and should not be more than an inch thick. You don't have to let everyone know what you are doing, just look at your palm and then at the meat. If it is too much, simply ask for a takeout container; and put the extra away for another meal. We are the ones in charge of what goes into our mouth, and it only takes a little while to learn something, which will aid in helping; to get the weight off. I know this was not something I picked up overnight, but with practice you too will begin to recognize the correct portion.

I was watching the television tonight, and they had a food eating contest on. Now I watched these three men, race to eat this enormous steak, and then sit back like it was natural. I wondered how many children watched the same show, and whether they now think, stuffing yourself like that is natural. I have three grandsons, and I teach them healthy eating habits. I don't want them to grow up and have to go through everything I have, just to get their weight in control; in order to save their lives. My three year old grandson will walk up to a stalk of broccoli, and dip it in his light ranch dressing, then he will remark "hummm...good to my stomach." If a child can learn to eat veggies, and think they are a treat; why can't an adult do it? We are what we know, knowledge is a wonderful thing. If you take time to learn the right way to do something, you enable yourself to succeed. Our relationship to food comes from how we have been raised, and how we live our lives. If all you are taught is fast food, you will find it difficult to adjust, but you can adjust with time. You didn't gain the weight overnight, and it's not going to disappear overnight. What you put into this is what you will get back out. Ask yourself are you ready to change? Am I ready to learn something new? Will I take a few changes in order to reach the goal of my dreams? If you said yes to any of these questions, then you are on the right road to success.

Embarrassing Moments

Many people say that they only want to forget their embarrassing moments, but I found that if you remember them, and laugh at them, that you are less likely to do the same thing over again. I thought I would give you a few moments which happen to me and I had to learn to live through them. Let's see where should I begin ... oh yes, there is no better place to start than at the Chicken Shack. I live in Michigan, and there is an eatery, which serves some of the best chicken; I have ever tasted. Well I went in one day, and my legs were hurting so bad that I decided to eat there instead of carrying it home. I went up to the counter like I had been doing for years, and placed my order, and quickly went and sat down. I told the young lady I would be eating in today, and she pointed to the silverware, and cups for the soda. Now I have been placing that order for 10 legs, 10 wings, 5 breasts, a large order of French fries and a large order of Cole slaw for years. When the order was ready, the waitress asked did I want her to bring a carry out container over. I looked at her in puzzlement; did she think I couldn't eat all of my food? I told her no, and I began to eat and eat. I hadn't noticed that while I was eating, the staffs of employees were all looking at me. They had no idea that I had been eating all of that food, by myself, all those years. I ate all but two pieces of chicken, and I probably would have eaten that, but I had drunk two 16 ounce cups of soda.

When it came time for me to leave, I asked the girl for another order of chicken, and French fries to go home with. The young girl looked at me her eyes said it all "are you sure?" she asked, then turned and went to place my order. The young man cleaning off the table smiled, and told me it had been interesting watching me eat. "Boy you can really shovel it in" he said as he cleaned off the table. "I was sure you couldn't eat that much food, but you sure fooled me!" I laughed, and told him that I was not feeling too hungry today, and he looked at me in amazement.

Now you see I told you this, so that you can see that overeating can become normal for anyone, who has a weight problem and haven't admitted it to them. I didn't care he saw me eating all that food, for I thought, it was a normal amount of food for me to consume. After all I was a big woman and it took a lot of food to fill me up. Why is it that we tend to think we need more to satisfy ourselves, when in truth we actually need less?

Now when I went to get up from that table, I want you to know, that the poor chair I was sitting on, had actually bent inwards. The manager came out and looked at the chair, gave me a stern look, then ordered the young man to take it into the back, and bring out another chair. I walked passed him picked up my order, and went to get into my car. It didn't matter to me, that when I got into my car; it would lean, and look like it was going to tip over. Yes, I had nerve to be riding in a little escort, and I would shove myself into that car like a sardine. Sound familiar? Oh yes, don't let me forget to tell you about the time I went to Kentucky Fried Chicken, and sat down on the bench, and it cracked from the pressure of my weight. I swore that it was defected, and that I should sue them, for the thing ripped my stocking. The manager quickly came around, and made sure I was okay; and told me the meal was on them. Boy had they made a mistake, I ordered two buckets of chicken, mash potatoes, Mac and cheese, Cole slaw, biscuits and honey. I even ordered some parfaits for dessert. When I left I heard someone say "boy she's got the biggest butt I have ever seen."

I have learned over the years to ignore the comments people make about my weight. I usually would get, "you have such a beautiful face", as the opening comment to their sentence (which usually ended with an insult). I never thought much about what they were saying about me once I left. Have you ever had a bench crack on you? How about chairs give way while you were sitting on it? Even worse was the time I sat down and ate, and got stuck in the booth. It took three staff members, and two male customers, to help me get out of the booth. Oh yes, I have some classic memories, that I have gone through, that I know many of you have experienced. I have gotten stuck in airplane seats, bathroom stalls at the mall, where I had trouble fitting through the door. These moments did not make me change, and trust me they won't make you change either. They were embarrassing alright, but they were a part of my life with the weight; and I considered them normal circumstances. Do you? Are you accepting those embarrassing moments as a normal part of your life?

Not all of my moments dealt with food, some of my classic moments, come through my children and grandchildren. I remember my second oldest grandchild, who at the time was four, telling his friends that I had two babies inside of my stomach. He just couldn't understand I wasn't pregnant, and that my weight was just that, *weight*. He would ask me to come out and play ball with him, and I would have good intentions, but after throwing one ball; I would tire, and tell him to go find something else to play with. I hated when I had to get up, and go and get the ball, which had rolled into an area, he was not permitted to go into. I would huff and puff my way to the ball, then would have to figure how I would get it. Often, I simply kicked it over to him; because I was unable to bend over, and pick it up. I have tons of memories of moments that I can't laugh at; but others have enjoyed laughing at me, and my greed. Have you been dismissing comments, rather than listening to them? Have embarrassing moments become almost natural to you? What will it take for you to change? Have you ever considered just what it would take for you to really change your life? Do you want to change but just don't know where to start? I did, so I began to research food; and just how long it takes for the food, I was consuming, to leave my body. It was hard for me to learn to carry measuring cups around, especially, hearing all of the comments, people were making around me. I remember I had been losing weight for about six months, when my grandson, one day turned to me and said, "Granny you look younger," he was beaming with a smile from ear to ear. He was proud of me, and this time he wasn't hiding his face, but standing there holding my hand. It never occurred to me, that he had been embarrassed to be with me. I thought nothing of the fat comments, people would make, but he did. A child of four, taught me that it does matter what people say, and I suddenly wasn't ashamed of taking out the cups, to measure my food; but proud to be doing it. I was learning how to succeed.

Success comes from learning how to succeed, and I was succeeding now. I was learning how to make it in this new life "one step at a time." I learned to laugh at myself, and I learned that I had to learn how to eat, all over again. Like a child, I had to adjust to eating food the right way. I complained, and fussed about the size amounts at first. "What do you mean my meat has to fit in the palm of my hand, and why can't it be more than an inch thick?" Have you ever experienced this thought before or something like it?

There are so many embarrassing moments in my life, that I could go on and on about them. I truly want the reader to know what I went through on this diet. I also want you to know what I have gone through after having bi-pass surgery. These are moments that I know you will understand and will consider what I am talking about. Thinking back now, I think the most embarrassing moment, for me, in my life; was when I was homeless and living in a shelter program. I became homeless in 2000 after I became severely ill, and had to stop working. I was self-employed so when I was unable to do my work, I soon found I could not pay, or maintain my bills. It was a very hard period in my life. I tell you this only because I want you to know why I gained forty pounds while staying in the shelter program. First and foremost, I want to thank the MCREST, rotating shelter program; this is a wonderful program. I was given thirty days under a roof; I wasn't sleeping on the streets. This was the thought, I took and held in my head all, through the program. I was a very large woman at 575 pounds. Losing my house sent me into a deep depression. I was just robbed, only several months before of everything of value. I was beside myself with grief. I couldn't just go get a job, I could barely walk. I had my pride, so I wouldn't tell my family how bad things were.

While in the program, they give you a thin mattress to sleep on. You can tell they care, because of all the means of comfort, they supply at night. The program makes everyone take a shower, before you can go to bed at night. It would have been no problem, only I weigh over five hundred pounds, and was ashamed to show my body, even if it was just to women. We all had to shower together, there were no private showers. So I had to undress and shower, then put my clothes on. It was horrible, I faced so many rude, and thoughtless comments, by the women. My heart, and spirit, was broken. I would shower and then go to dinner. You could eat as much as you wanted, after everyone was fed. Because of my size, I had to have help lying down on my mattress, I had to have help getting up off the mattress; (it took three women to pull me up off the floor.) I would go to dinner, and stuff myself, I would eat, two to three plates of food. I would take two lunches, one to eat when I got to the Mall and one to eat for lunch. During this month, I went through so much humiliation, that I simply at to cover my sadness. I was eating enough food, for three or four people. When I finally was able to get an apartment I had gain 37.7 pounds.

Getting the apartment meant that I was improving but it didn't feel like it. I was only able to find a one bedroom with a kitchen and full bath; the apartment was beautiful, only it was upstairs and I had to climb ten stairs to get to it. I would huff and puff my way up and down those stairs and would often have to sit on the landing and catch my breath. I had a friend from the shelter to come and help me with my housekeeping. I thought I was doing well. I had transportation solved by the bus picking me up. I would have to climb the two stairs to get into the bus. I would sometimes take 5 minutes to just get into the bus. When my housekeeper got sick and had to leave, I was unable to find a replacement. I had an accident when I fell down the stairs trying to take the garbage out. I had to move and all of it became a mess. I was eating so much during this period I found myself unable to stop eating I had to have the food. It was as though the food was giving me some kind of a fix. I believe and know now that food can be like a drug; and for many like me they survive on eating.

I was having difficulty walking, climbing stairs, and even in taking care of myself. For my hands, had developed copper tunnel, and I could barely feel my fingers. I ate to make myself feel better. I ate to hide how sad I was, this period was devastating, for me to live through. I can't say I didn't learn from the experience, I can say I say what depression and sadness can do, to a person who is an overeater, or hides their problems in eating. I was one of these people. I was embarrassed and so I ate, and ate. Have you been through some moments, which were so embarrassing? That you ate your way through them? Can you understand now that you have only made the problem worse? Food is meant to nourish us, and true it gives us pleasure; but if you cannot control your own eating, and if you are gaining weight; maybe you need to consider such as I did, that a change had to be made.

Just because you find yourself ready to make a change doesn't mean that you will be willing to adjust to the changes as they come. You have to learn to move forward and be willing to accept the necessary changes. One is that you have to learn to eat properly. You need to know when you are over eating or when you are really hungry. These things come with time and knowledge as you begin to pick up the pieces and start accepting the program. You will have to buy the set of measuring cups and look at them as a way of growing. You will grow thinner as you use them, and more important; you will begin to understand how to eat the right amount of food. We need to learn in order to grow, and I hope that as you read this book, you will pick up your measuring cups; and begin to grow into the person you want to be. You may not have to lose a pound, but you still will learn correct proportion, and that's the goal of this book.

You will be a success for you will learn just how to do it. I have lost on my own, by learning how to eat over 348 pounds, and I hope that you too, will be able to say I have lost a few pounds. Whether you have to lose 2 or 2000 you will be able to do it! We have everything to live for, and we have every right to have respect, for what we accomplish, in our effort to reach our goals. So sit back and relax, and learn. Welcome to "What Weight!!" you're about to become a new person, one that you will love. More important, you will be able to help someone else, get through the same problems you had; and show them the correct way to succeed. Life is a learning process, and even when it comes to the illness of overeating; one needs to learn how to overcome the habit of eating too much, and allow themselves a chance to heal. Overeating is an illness, like cancer it can kill you. With treatment there is a chance that you will heal and survive, and one day reach your goal. Remember that when you make your decision, to change your life; you will have to make new choices, many you will make but it will take time for you to accept them.

How to Really Get Started Accepting Yourself

There is no miracle drug, or cure that will help you; with the step that is the most important, when it comes to succeeding...truth. It takes truth, in accepting that you need to change your life, and your lifestyle. It is not an easy thing facing oneself. You would think you could just look in the mirror, and say okay this is me, and I'm going to love myself, and that would be that. No way! I come to tell you that the hardest thing, in the world for me, was to look into a full length mirror, naked at my own body. I just couldn't see myself; it hurt so much to see my body, a mass of lumps of fat. I had breasts that were measuring in at 54 inches, and the midsection of my body was 48 inches, and my hips were 168 inches wide. I tell you this, not in pride, but in truth; for I want you to realize, that I was no beauty queen. I was a woman who had eaten, and over the years put on 495lbs. I remember going to Receiving Hospital, for severe pain in my back and legs. When they asked my weight, I didn't have any idea. I was too heavy for all of the scales they had, so they had to call for this scale they weighed cargo on, to get my accurate weight. I thought I would die, getting up on that scale; and when the dials weigh me in at 495.7 pounds, I truly thought I would just die. I looked around at the nurses and the man walking down the hall; and got off the scale in embarrassment, and walked back to my room with the assistance of the nurse. I knew then I had to do something, and for you, I pray it won't take something, so dramatic, to help you make, and take the courage, to change your life.

I didn't change right away. I kept eating the food, I was adjusted to. I was eating a little less, like instead of two plates of chicken wings I ate one. I want the reader, to understand that proportion, is so important. If you want to master good health, and good eating habits; you first have to learn what the correct proportion eating really is, and how to use it in your life. I was eating the correct foods, but I was overeating to the point, I was gaining instead of losing. So once you have mastered looking into the mirror, at your body, and accepting that you need to make changes. I want you to accept that you can do it, that you can look into your inner soul, and accept yourself, and that you are ready; to make the move towards good healthy living. Look at every angle of your body, that's important; for you have to know what you have to work on. I know that it will be hard to do; it took everything in me, to look at myself sideways. I looked like a big round blimp. I had never looked at my body naked, and especially sideways. I nearly fainted at what I looked like. I know it will be hard, but you must do it; for you have to look at yourself, and accept yourself, before you can make the changes; that will help you succeed, in what you are really want, and that is becoming a healthier and happier person.

Healthy eating is what I am going to teach you; but more important, as you read, you will begin to feel better about yourself, and you will have more **knowledge, about food, and how it affects your bodies. I want you to grow in** knowledge, for that is what will help you succeed. When you don't know the right proportions, you over eat, and harm yourself. I found that when I learned what the right proportion was, I was feeling at first, like I was going to starve, eating so little. The truth of the matter is that at first you do feel a little hungry. I found a way to get through that, by eating healthy snacks. I have the meal, and true; it has to taste good, but sometimes, I might feel a little hungry, about a half hour later. So I had to learn to find things to eat, which would not put the pounds on me, but would help me to lose weight. I love to nibble, and if you are a nibbler, you will find that I have some great tips for you. If you are someone who loves to feel full, you will find that this healthy eating can succeed even for you; for you will feel full, and satisfied. Have you looked into the mirror yet? Have you looked at yourself sideways, and now know what areas of your body, you need to improve? Are you okay? Did you have a hard time doing it, or was it easy for you to accept, the areas that needed to be improved on? If you are ready, and I mean when you are ready, then you will be ready to live a healthy life. Nothing will happen overnight, but as you read you begin to adjust to what you know is the truth. These adjustments are what make us stronger in the long run. I found that I because much stronger in all areas of my life, once I had gotten hold of my eating problems and began to change them. It doesn't take a master mind, or a learned teacher, to show one how to make the steps necessary for changing their lives. What it does take is the power and the ability to accept and put into action the things that you learn. The first step is learning proportion in relation to food, so let's get started.

THE FIRST THING YOU HAVE TO DO IS BUY YOURSELF A SET OF MEASURING CUPS! THESE CUPS WILL BECOME YOUR BEST FRIEND OVER THE NEXT FEW WEEKS!!

To succeed, all you have to do; is learn how much of each food, you can consume, and burn off that day. I could barely walk, when I started measuring my food. I didn't like the small amounts at first. I kept doing it, and soon I began to see; that I knew the size amount, and didn't need the cup. I also want you to get a small saucer, one that is used for coffee, would be great. This plate is what you will measure your meat on, and you will find, it will hold up to four ounces. This will help you, with the control; you will need, with meat, and also teach you proportion; which will help, in making you healthier. For instance I use to eat a medium size bowl, of grits, with 2 tablespoons of butter; 3eggs, with ½ cup of cheese, mixed in them. 4 strips of bacon, and sometimes 5 link sausages, for breakfast. I left off the fact; I ate 3-4 slices of rye bread, toasted and buttered; coffee, with 4-5 sugars, and cream. I usually would drink 3 cups of coffee. Now this was my breakfast, and I ate it every day, for over thirty years. Changing my eating habits was no easy task for me. I had to learn to let go of my bad eating habits. Letting go is hard, but it can be done, It ***Because I did.***

I wish I could make you accept, the simple truth about good health, but it's hard to explain. Once you learn how to eat, and the proper amount of food, which is acceptable as normal; you will find yourself, understanding, and the weight, will begin to drop off quickly. I couldn't lose a thing at first, it wasn't because I didn't cook the food right, or even, that I wasn't watching what I ate; I simply was overeating, mainly because, I had no idea what size proportion was; and it was hurting me. The old saying, "what you don't know, won't hurt you, is bull!!" I was eating myself, to an early grave, simply because I was overeating. It was not easy for me to accept, the right portion size; I felt I was going to starve. I had already brainwashed myself, into believing, that I was not going to be able to do it. So the first step for me, was accepting the fact, I was overeating, and learning what the correct portion was, for each item I was eating. Once you know how much, you can eat of an item, you can also judge, how much you are over eating. There are many things, which we eat, that we can indulge ourselves, and it will not hurt us. While there are others, which if we take one bite too much, we have pounds, on the hips to show for it. So grab a set of measuring cups, take time to find a set that you like, for you will be using them every day, for the next few months. It took me three months, before I was able to know, and recognize the size portion for my food. I remember I was sitting in a restaurant, with my friend, when I told him that I had entirely too much food, on my plate. I signaled for the waitress, and asked for a takeout container. I put the extra food, in the container, and I still had a plate full, of food to enjoy, with my friend. He was impressed to see, that I had gotten control, of my overeating. I was proud of myself, and at the end of three months, the scale showed the results, I had lost seventeen pounds; and came down two dress sizes. I can't believe that I owe it to measuring cups!!!

If you find you need more time, to practice using the cups, and learning the food charts and amounts, it's okay. I often go back, and review, my charts and amounts; because it's so important. I don't need to eat, French fries for two, anymore, I can settle on half and order. I can enjoy a grilled hamburger (try turkey, chicken and pork have the butcher ground it fresh for you) and still lose weight. Healthy eating is good for your whole body, and it's only helping you excel, in your goals. I didn't lose weight overnight, it took me three years. One and a half years, were spent learning; how to eat healthy, and learning the proper amounts. I made many mistakes, and had to start over time after time, but I began to learn, and the pounds began to shed off of me. I can't express it enough, when it comes to learning, how to be healthy, it is a one step at a time process. You will learn and the cups will no longer be necessary, for you to carry around; but until that day, those cups, are going to be your best friend. You will carry them everywhere, and you will not mind, pulling them out, and filling them up. My friends, and many people watching me, using them asked; what I was doing, and once I told them, and they saw how much food, they were overeating, they started using the cups; to help them learn, to eat healthy. Healthy eating, leads to a healthy body, and that leads to a longer, and more productive life.

Remember the cups, are great for some items, but when it comes to meat you need a different measurement.

You need to get a coffee saucer, and learn to measure your meat, to fit the plate. Only remember the meat, should not be more, than one to two inches, in thickness. It's not the meat, which causes the problem, it's the fact, and we don't know the correct amount, of the meat to eat. We are definitely, a society of people, who have been raised, to overeat. Strange, in a world where, there is so much hunger, and starvation; we suffer from over indulgence. I use to use the tip of my finger, to measure my meat, and that way, I never was too far off base. The size of the plate is the same size, as the palm of your hand, and you should never consume more, than the palm can hold. I hope you will at least try my idea for thirty days, and see if you adjust, or notice a change. Sometimes, it's not the weight ,that's important, maybe you; didn't lose a pound, but then your blood pressure dropped, that's an accomplishment; and you should give yourself a hug, it's a sign, that the effort, you are putting forth, to learn good healthy habits, is paying off.

So over the next few weeks, you will be learning some new techniques, to help you, in reaching your goals. I hope that you will give yourself the time, to learn them, and remember, ***"GETTING** HEALTHY, IS AS SIMPLE, AS LEARNING TO TAKE IT, ONE STEP AT A TIME!! YOU HAVE ALREADY MADE THE FIRST STEP, YOU READ THIS CHAPTER!! GOOD LUCK WITH YOUR CUPS!!!!*

CUPS CAN BE EMBRASSING!

I could pretend and tell you, that I was never embarrassed; using my cups, but that would be an absolute lie. I was plenty embarrassed, at first when I started using them, and you will be embarrassed too, don't fool yourself. Food is to be enjoyed and to truly do that, one must not be afraid, of the food. Fear is dangerous, especially, for those who have to lose, or monitor their weight. Somehow knowing you have to monitor, or weigh food, before you eat; you cause the mind to turn to fear. Fear, can be as simple, as not knowing, how much of an item; one can consume, to as severe as overeating, and causing yourself serious health problems. To concur fear, all one has to do, is simply face it head on. When it comes to food, it is necessary, to know how to cook it, and how much of it, can you consume. More important, what must I do, in burning those calories off, to keep my weight, at a healthy level? So food and exercise go together, and as you learn, the **amounts** which are healthy, you will also learn, what you have to do to burn that off, and that way, you will begin to not only concur, the fear of food, but find yourself getting healthier.

One of my most precious moments, was when I was out with my youngest grandson, and we stopped to eat. When the food came, he looked up, and said "Granny no Cups!" I smiled for him, it was normal to see me, pull out the cups, and measure my food. Suddenly, I knew I was going to make it, and you will too! The power to control, is within the mind, and so if one learns, the what (amount), and how (much) of an item, or food, they assume the control. You can't expect to lose weight, and keep it off, if you don't take time, to learn how to match, what you eat in activity. I said ACTIVITY, because I learned there are many ways to burn calories. Some are as simple as reading a book, to raking the leaves out of the yard. But I found the best way, to burn calories, is in walking, and outdoor exercises. There is power in nature, and if you find a good walking trail, at a park, you can enjoy the smells, and sounds of the earth, as you walk away the pounds.

Putting the amounts of the food, in your head, and matching it with what amount of exercise, you have to burn off, is power. I learned that if I wanted to eat, a cup of rice, a cup of greens, 4 ounces of chicken, along with one cup of lettuce, for dinner; that I had to walk, three miles, to burn off the calories. This was important to me, for I wanted to be able, to eat and enjoy my food, and not worry, about gaining weight. You will begin to match food, and exercise, in your head, and you too, will see the pounds, began to fall off. More than that, you will find that with the lost of pounds, comes a feeling of pride, because you have mastered the power of fear, when it comes to eating.

Once again I stress the importance of learning, the amounts; you can't do that any simpler, than carrying a measuring cup. I found all you need, is the regular plastic measuring cup, in your hand, and you can control any food. I also learned, that I can't eat a cup, of most food, that I am a ½ cup person. I can eat 3, and sometimes 4 ½ ounces of meat, at a time. So I can consume 2 cups of food, at a time. To know how much it takes to fill you up is important, for it controls, whether you overeat. If you want to eat a burger with fries, you need to include everything, which makes that possible. Can you lose without measuring, or exercise? Sure, but you will gain it back. It has been proven with research, that people who lose weight quickly, or even with surgery, they don't succeed as well, as those they researched, that learn to weigh, and eat healthy, but also did exercise. There is much, much more, that goes with losing weight, than you think. What you eat is important, as well as the scenery, and how you react to it. What we see, and what we smell, goes with what we eat, or don't eat.

To lose weight, one must first, learn the basics to our bodies. Everything is different, and no two people, are the same. Weight is different, in each person's body, and so is the plan, which will jump start, their weight loss. It doesn't matter if you have to lose 5 pounds, or 500, you need to learn, just what your body needs. For most of us, it will take determination, and courage, to start the diet, and succeed; but to do so; you first have, to follow some simple steps.

Accept the truth that you need to make a step, to learn how to eat healthy. Did you notice, I didn't mention the word, diet? YOU, have to decide, to eat healthy. Once you have done that, you will find the next step to easy. Healthy eating, will automatically lead, to weight and said she had learned anything can happen. She made me realize, that I had to do something, about my overeating, and learn more, about how to get control. I am not one, for making changes. I hate rushing. I like to do things, slow and easy, when it comes to life now. I guess that's why, it was so hard for me, at first, I didn't really want to change, but change, is what is needed, if you are going, to succeed. I hope I can get you, to understand ,just how important, it means learning, what proportion is, and why it is going to be, the most important thing, in your life, the next few months. It takes time to learn, to rethink, not only your way of eating, but also learning, how to put exercise, into your life. It is easy to say, but harder to do, but if you take things, one step at a time, then you will succeed.

My evening with my friend, was cut short, I often couldn't blame him, when I think back. I was so uncomfortable, I was scared to eat. I felt like everyone, was sitting around, waiting for my pants, to rip again. It was a terrible date, and I often wished I could have had the chance, to go out with him again. I found out a year ago, that he had a stroke, standing in the line, at the bank. He never got a chance, to even fight, his body was weak, and he lacked proper nutrition. He was good, at exercising, but bad at eating, and so he lacked nutrition. Here I thought, he was perfect, and he showed me, that he had need of, as much help, as I, myself did. The power of change, comes from inside the heart, and is transferred to the brain. I believe this statement is true, for everyone; first you must accept the truth, in order to proceed to the next step, which is achieving the goal. You accept the truth, in your heart, first, and foremost. This truth could be as simple, as the fact, you are hungry, to the truth and acceptance, that you must seek help, in reaching your goal. The heart is where the door of entrance begins, but the brain, is where the knowledge is stored.

To reach any goal, or make any movement, one must want, or need something. From birth, one has a need, or wants for something; such as a need for love, or hunger, and a need for someone, to feed us, or give us, that love. We seek knowledge from birth, and that fact is important, because of how the knowledge, is given to us, and how we receive it. If you need love, and get hatred, or pain, you accept that knowledge, as a truth. This is dangerous, look at how children, and adults, react when they have been abused, or not given proper love?

The first thing you have to do is to learn what your truth is. Do you need to lose a few pounds? Maybe you need to learn how to eat, all over again, after all, for many Diabetics, this is a truth. They learn they have diabetes, and that they have to learn how, to eat all over again. It is a hard truth, that doesn't come easy. For many people, changing their eating style will not only be hard, but at times very insulting. I remember a friend, who found out they had diabetes, and that they would now, have to eat differently. It didn't matter to her, that she was putting her, life in danger; she didn't want to change anything. She was defeated at the start, because she conditions herself, to believe that she couldn't do it. Are you like her? Are you already telling yourself, that you will fail? Let me tell you a truth, which you will find hard to accept, but will as the months go by. YOU CAN DO IT!!!

At 575lbs. I thought after numerous diets that failed, that I could not stick to a diet plan. Well I could, once I stopped calling it a diet, and started simply saying, "I'm learning to eat healthy." The mind is a funny thing, it will accept whatever, you teach it, with time. I first had to learn, how to eat healthy, and for me, that was difficult. For I had spent most of my life eating unhealthy. I lived on hamburgers, and fries, and shakes, and for the most part, Beef was my main meat. When I found out how long it takes Beef, to leave the body (three days), I began to add up, just how much harm, I was doing to myself. You see I ate a burger nearly every day, and I calculated that it was taking two weeks, to get the burgers, from one week, out of me. I had never considered, while I was eating, that I was hurting, myself, so when I finally, took hold of the situation, I had a month of burgers, to get rid of. It took me nearly two months, of waiting, to get the beef, out of my system, before I could even start watching, to see if the new menu, I was eating was working or not. So if you are a beef eater, then I suggest, you do what I did, and put beef, out of your diet, for a few months. Did you notice, I didn't say stop, eating beef. I enjoy eating a beef burger, at least once a month, the rest of the month; I focus on turkey burger, veggie burgers and chicken burgers. I have found so many ways to make burgers that are healthy, that I truly don't miss the beef. So the statement "where's the beef?" can be answered, in the fridge, and not on my hips.

I found that there are many ways, to enjoy meat, and its fun learning, how to enjoy food, that doesn't come from a cow. I want you to understand, if you are a beef eater, you only have to control it, not stop eating it. Learning how to balance, your diet is important, that means learning how to incorporate fruit, and vegetables; as well, as starch, into your eating habits, is necessary. I thought, I would be hungry, but the truth of the matter, was that I was eating more, and losing more, with each passing day. It takes time to learn, how to eat, so don't fool yourself; it will take time, for you also to learn. After all, you wouldn't have to lose anything, if you were doing it right, from the beginning, but like most of us, you learned to eat wrong, and have to retrain yourself, to eat correctly. I don't have any miracles, or miracle drugs, to tell you about, but I do have solutions, to problems that most of us, encounter, and ways that you can work, your way through them.

Learning to eat your way thin is the most enjoyable way of losing weight, I have found. No matter whether you have to lose one pound, or 300, when you learn to eat correctly, and learn portion control, you will find that you have given, yourself the start that you need to succeed. I decided that as with any self help book, the content, must be one that you can follow. So to help you get a hand on it, I have included breakfast, lunch, and dinner; as well as snacks in a program, which you pick and chose. No one likes the same thing every day, and all of us, like to feel, we have control, of what we want to eat. Learning to eat healthy, is easy, it's the trial period, which takes a little time. Sure you will need a period of readjusting, but it's an adjustment, that you can get use to. As with any new diet plan, or change, I recommend you check, with your doctor, to see whether, it will be safe for you, to start.

Once given the go ahead, then look over the menus, and find the ones, which appeal to you, then make your grocery list, and get started. To ensure your success, I recommend you clean house, by getting rid of anything, which will cause you to cheat. I have grandchildren, and I first used the excuse, that I had to have chips, and cookies etc., in the house for them. The truth of the matter was, I was wrong, my grandchildren, loved eating my food, and they found, pleasure in trying out the new things. I remember when I made my first batch of sugar free cookies, and tried it out on them. They loved the cookies, they didn't know they were sugar free, they thought they were eating regular cookies, and I left it at that. In fact my three year old grandson often says "hummm…good to my stomach" every time he eats vegetables. I remember when I first started showing him how to dip his vegetables, into my low fat dip. He smiled and said "hummmm." He learned to eat healthy, from watching me eat, and to him it's normal. You see he wasn't told, it's a diet, or that it's different, only that it was good. You will learn that even for you, and your family, if you don't mention its low fat, or reduced calorie, that they will simply enjoy eating something new. Remember, we are taught to enjoy food, and so teach them to enjoy eating healthy, it's something which will make all of you smile. I have menus for teens, as well as, for office a worker, taking a lunch, is taken to a new plateau and you will find everyone, in the family reap its rewards.

So grab your measuring cups and plates, and let's get ready to eat our way, to a healthier and longer life. Remember that all you have to do, is stick to the format, so before you begin take time, to look over all of the menus, and decided which ones you want to try out first. You have to eat every four hours, often you will fill full, but eat anyway. Do not miss a meal, or change the format, because it will only cause you to cheat. The menus have been based off of a low income budget, so that anyone can follow them. Low budget, doesn't mean low taste, you learn to use spices and seasoning, which bring out the flavor of the food. If a food doesn't have enough flavors then try adding something else to flavor it. I found that most foods can be doctored up, to taste enjoyable to you, with trial and error. In all cooking, and formation, of menus you should try adding dried or either fresh herbs, to boost the flavor.

Herbs, add a different touch to meats, veggies and fruits but remember when using dried herbs, and fruits, not to overdo. Fresh herbs, are my herbs of choice, I find that I enjoy the flavor, as well as the color it adds, to the meal. But even fresh herbs, can overpower a dish, if too much is added, once again trial and error, is what is needed. Not to waste the food, why not try adding a little at a time, until you get to the desired taste you enjoy. For those who are diabetic, you will find most of the menus, are acceptable. Diabetes must maintain control of their food, but the principals, with which the program works, on can be used even for them. You see it is the amount of the foods; you are eating, which will hold the clue, to your success. I cannot stress enough, the importance of measuring what you eat. I am not a dietitian, but I have been using diets, in one way or the other, for over thirty plus years; the following guideline, is what I formed, to follow at the beginning of my weight loss and after trying it out on numerous people found it works on just about everyone. It is once again the amount of the food, which is important, if you keep to the amounts, you will find yourself, not only losing but slowly gaining control, of your eating.

BREAKFAST
(This meal should never be skipped
and can be eaten at anytime)

3 oz of meat or 1 egg
1 cup of fresh fruit
1 slice of bread or ½ c. cereal
4 oz of non-fat or skim milk

This breakfast menu will not only give you nutrients but will give you the energy boost needed to jump start your day. Eggs should be monitored and should not be eaten for breakfast every day. Diabetics should remember that all fruit changes to sugar in the body so they should monitor themselves. Bi-pass surgery patient should add the powdered protein to their skim milk or soy milk. Also of importance is the fact that something should be eaten every three hours. This will eliminate, the hunger feeling, which over takes the body, in between meals. Snacks, are consumed in between each meal, and should not be omitted. They help us control hunger, and help to keep that empty feeling out of the stomach. Please keep in mind that you should check with your doctor, to see if you can follow the plan which I used to get rid of my weight.

You should also keep in mind that you should be starting a daily routine for yourself, when it comes to exercise both inside and outdoors. I did some things indoors at first, only because of my size and the fact I was unable to do them outdoors. I had a great deal of trouble moving around, but I know that if you work out even just a little that it helps in keeping the muscles from sagging. I wish I had started tightening my muscles earlier than what I did; I would not have some of the problems I have now with my thighs and arms. Of importance is the fact that you have to accept that exercise and food go together. What I eat I have to burn off…if not instead of losing, you will find yourself gaining. I started this diet many times before I finally starting following it. I didn't lose anything when I played at losing, it wasn't until I started following the program, reading the material, and following the recipes, that the weight soon started coming off.

Snacks are important. They help you keep on track when you are monitoring your weight or food portions. I found that legal snacks not only helped me what they saved my life many a day. On those days that I was really stressed out, I would eat legal snacks instead of potato chips, cookies, etc. They kept me from gaining and also kept me from overeating. I hope that some of my favorites will be yours too. I once again say check with your doctor to make sure that you can have the snacks I have listed. The amounts were what I came to adjust to and still follow. I lost my weight, went through the maintence program, and now maintain my weight all from the same foods. I didn't have to change or readjust to anything again because this program is a healthy one and it is meant to be followed for life. I enjoy cookies, cakes, and doughnuts even now but I make them myself and I use a sugar substitute and keep to the normal serving size. I have even learned to make my own low fat ice cream. It's fun to do and can be made to be a fun family evening.

SNACKS

1 cup fruit
1 cup vegetables
1 starch (can be 1 slice of bread or five crackers)
1 oz of dairy (can be yogurt or cheese)
1 bowl of shredded lettuce with 1 tablespoon of low calorie dressing
1 cup of cubed gelatin (I like mixing ½ cup of fruit inside)
Coffee, tea, or diet soda (8 ounces only)

No meat should be eaten during snack time the only time meat is consumed is during the basic meal. There are many reasons for this, but the one I want you to remember is that, you are retraining yourself to eat healthy. Healthy eating will lead to a healthy body. Isn't that what it is really all about? You want to eat to live, but you also want to eat to enjoy yourself. I stuck to this snack program, substituting where necessary to keep from getting bored. Bi-pass patients can add powdered protein to their dairy. I chose to use strawberry protein mix, mainly because it mixes well with all kinds of fruit. Also the protein is needed in restoring the muscles to normal. Diabetics might need to cut ½ of the fruit down, make sure you check with your doctor, before starting this diet plan.

LUNCH

3 oz of meat
1 cup of vegetables
1 cup of fruit
1 starch
1 calcium
1 small bowl of shredded lettuce with dressing
Coffee, tea, diet soda

After any meal even snacks water should be consumed and this should not be mistaken for diet sodas, coffee or tea. Liquid refreshments are added liquids and should be monitored but not within the meal itself. A good tip is to drink liquids after the meal and not during. The water or liquid will confuse you and make you feel you are full but as with all liquids which the body consumes they wear off and you will be left with a desire to eat. I found drinking the water or pop etc. after the main food has been consume easier and that the control of the amounts were easier to handle and stick to. If you feel full you must still eat what is required the success of the diet itself depends on you eating all of the food even snacks every three hours. Before the bi-pass surgery the food on the plan would keep me satisfied. I wouldn't cheat because there was so much food to eat. I find that that is still true even with the surgery. I get full with the meal and my drink and it still takes me time to consume the food. The good thing about the program I followed was just how I was able to feel full when I ate. This full feeling helped me stay focus and on the program.

A good tip to remember is if in between the meals and snacks you are still hungry then try eating a small salad with a low calorie diet dressing. Drink a glass of flavored water with a slice of fruit inside. This will fill you and give you the added boost needed to stick to the program. I do suggest that you try spring greens instead of iceberg lettuce. Spring greens stay fresher longer and contain more nutrients than regular lettuce. I like putting fresh herbs inside of my salads they add another level of flavor to the salad. I found that if I was extremely hungry I would add thin sliced fresh fruit to the top of the salad greens. This gives variety and also gives flavor which is important. When adding herbs to my salads my favorite is adding basil or parsley to the greens its effect is amazing and the added taste helps control the appetite.

There were many things that you can combine from off the snack chart; you simply have to take time not to over eat an item. If you want a potato you can have it but it should be a cup of potatoes. You have to learn to measure your food in order to gain control of your eating. You need to know if an item is to be eaten as much as you like or if you have to watch your intake of that item. You will find that it won't take long for you to adjust. You will enjoy the amount of food and soon adjust to the way the program works.

Adjustment has to be made and if you take time to pull your efforts together properly by learning what to do you will succeed. You can't expect to climb the mountain unless you are willing to use the gear. It takes time and sometimes determination to reach your goal. I have faith that I was going to will and I would not let anything or anyone change my mind. It might take that for you, are you ready to reach higher?

DINNER

3oz of meat
2 cups of vegetables
1 cup of fruit
1 starch
1 calcium
1 cup of shredded lettuce or spring greens
1 low calorie dessert
Coffee, tea, or diet soda (remember when it comes to diet sodas or drinks only consume 8 ounces)
1 small bowl of chicken broth with herbs

Notice the change in the vegetables for dinner and also notice that the salad in this meal is included inside of the meal. Dinner should always come with a salad and I started each meal with a cup of broth which had fresh herbs floating on top. The following is the method of making the broth which should be consumed and also can be used for cooking purposes. Salt should not be added to any of the food but if you use salt remember to monitor its use, or use a salt substitute. I couldn't find a salt substitute I liked so I just stuck to using less and less salt.

HOMEMADE CHICKEN BROTH

1 WHOLE CHICKEN CUT AND QUARTERED
1 teaspoon dried basil

1 teaspoon thyme
1 teaspoon rosemary
2 teaspoons minced garlic
2 teaspoons dehydrated onions (can be omitted)
1 carrot sliced thin

Place washed chicken into a pot and cover with water and add seasoning then bring the chicken to a rapid boil for fifteen minutes then turn off and cover. Let stand for 1 hour and remove the chicken which can be cooked and used later. The broth should be placed in storage containers and froze for future use. I like using single use containers for storing so that if needed I didn't have to waste the broth itself. Remember to skim the fat off the top of the cooled broth and discard it before storing the mixture. I also make a broth from ham bones and beef steak bones using the same method. The ham and steak bone broth is a delightful change and helps to keep you focus on the diet. Broth can be consumed in between the meals with snacks with a salad to help control hunger but the regular snack menu should be followed at all times. As you see there is a large amount of food which is consumed during the course of the day. Remember with this diet you are eating your way thin and the more you eat the more you lose.

ALL MEAT SHOULD BE BAKED, BROILED, BOILED OR GRILLED. FRIED FOODS ARE ONLY PERMITTED IF THEY ARE OVEN FRIED.

All fried food should be drained on paper towels so that excess oil can be removed from the food before consuming. The following homemade dressings can be used to dress up a salad and can be used on meat as a flavor change.

Yogurt Dressing
(Ranch substitute)

8oz plain yogurt
¼ c skim milk
1 packet ranch dressing
1 teaspoon lemon juice

Mix ingredients well before adding lemon juice. To spike up the taste try adding
¼ teaspoon dried parsley
¼ teaspoon dried basil
½ teaspoon onion powder
½ teaspoon garlic powder
2 Tablespoon light olive oil

Store dressing for three days in air tight container. Shake or mix well before using. Try serving over spring greens, fresh baby spinach with shredded carrots. Leave out the milk and lemon juice and serve with homemade baked pita chips or tortilla strips (which have been baked in the oven)

Homemade pita or tortilla chips

Use a whole wheat pita or tortilla. You can even use a tomato or spinach flavored one for variety. Cut into squares or diamonds for pita bread. And for the chips make them about ½ inches thick. Spray with non stick cooking spray and bake in a preheated oven 400 degrees for about ten minutes or until crisp. When they come out of the oven spray again with a non stick spray and sprinkle with your favorite seasonings. Let cool before handling they are extremely hot.

Zesty Italian Dressing

¾ cup light olive oil
¼ cup of apple cider vinegar
1 Tablespoon dried Italian seasoning
¼ teaspoon thyme
¼ teaspoon onion powder
¼ teaspoon garlic powder
Pinch of pepper flakes
¼ teaspoon black pepper

Blend well and store in air tight container for up to a week. Serve over fresh greens but for a change of pace try marinating chicken or pork for thirty minutes then grilling. Try serving over thinly sliced red onions, tomatoes and cucumbers and top with thinly chopped fresh basil

French Made Easy

½ cup tomato sauce
¼ cup light olive oil
3 Tablespoon apple cider vinegar
2 Tablespoon evaporated skim milk
¼ teaspoon dried basil
1 teaspoon low calorie sweetener

Mix well and store in air tight container for three days. Serve over fresh spinach or for a change of pace add thin slice apples and toasted walnuts or almonds. Try baking chicken thighs for 40 minutes in the dressing let cool before serving over ½ cup of rice

Sweet and Spicy Dressing

1 cup of light olive oil
1/4 cup apple cider vinegar
Red pepper flakes to taste
3 teaspoons diet sweetener of choice
¼ teaspoon garlic powder
¼ teaspoon onion powder
¼ teaspoon black pepper

Mix well keep in air tight container for 3-4 days. Try serving this dressing over a thinly sliced apple and red onion salad. Add a little color by sectioning an orange and adding a few of the slices. Try marinating chicken wing dings in the dressing overnight and grilling them and drizzling a little dressing (which has been reduced on the stove) on the wings before serving them.

Most marinades can be reduced on the stove or grill to kill bacteria but also to make a sauce to pour over the meat or salad before serving. Make sure to heat the marinade thoroughly on a low heat so that all of the bacteria are killed. Most reductions take ten to fifteen minutes so don't rush them. Many the recipes have been changed in order to improve the flavor. I hope that if you don't like something you will try to doctor it up by changing the flavor or herbs to suit you. The portion must stay the same, remember you can only consume meat at main meals and meat should never be more than three to four ounces at a serving.

The one thing I have learned on this diet is that meat takes a long time to leave the body. That is why I do not include meat in the snacks, but there are exceptions to this. I eat peanut butter, sardines, mussels, oysters, when it comes to snacks. I am a bariatric patient and I have to consume a lot of protein. This helps the muscles and it also helps with the hunger. I hope that the reader will consider such as I did, that meat should be limited. I do not list my recipes in this book for a reason; I want you to browse through them. If you know where something is you will limit yourself to one item. In browsing you will find that you might want to change what you are looking for to something else. For instance, I wanted to eat chicken one day, so I went browsing through my recipes. I found one for stuffed cabbage made with bean sprouts. I can't tell you how good that stuff cabbage was and I would have never tried it if I hadn't been browsing through the recipes. I don't want you to become to settled, it's not good when you are trying to lose weight. You need to browse and look and see just what will satisfy you and when you do then you will find that you are happier with your choice.

QUESTIONS AND ANWSERS

1. **Should I seek medical advice before starting this program?**

   Yes. With any new adventure you should seek medical advice before starting. It's important to know whether or not you are diabetic, have heart problems etc. Your doctor will advise you on whether the program would be good for you. Most doctors approve the program especially when they see you are willing to follow it.

2. **Is hunger a major issue in your program?**

   No, Most will find that they have to carry over the food to the next meal they are just too full. It is important to eat all of the food listed so that you can follow the program and achieve success. Failure comes from trying to cut the amounts down, you leave yourself open to feeling hunger and if that happens defeat will soon follow.

3. **Do you have to use the measuring cups when fixing your plate?**

> Yes. Using the measuring cups help you to learn control and portion control is very important when it comes to success. I do not recommend trying to follow the program without the cups they help you not to overeat as well. **Don't underestimate the power of the measuring cup when it comes to success.**

4. **Can dry herbs and spices be used in place of the fresh herbs? Aren't fresh herbs expensive?**

> Yes, dry herbs and spices can replace the fresh herbs but you use less since it's more potent. No, fresh herbs are expensive when you consider the flavor they add to the meal. Fresh herbs can be air dried and then placed in zip lock bags and frozen. You can also freeze fresh herbs and use them right out of the freezer when cooking. The flavor is far better than dried and you taste the herb even better when compared with dried herbs. With dry herbs you use less because it is potent and you down want to overpower the flavor within the meal.

5. **I am on a limited budget will I be able to afford the food to do this program?**

> Yes. The pride of this program is the fact that it was designed around the "Save-A-Lot" budget. Fresh fruit can be substituted with can fruit but use the sugar free or light fruit and run the fruit under cool water before serving and

make sure it is chilled before eating. Fresh or frozen vegetables are recommended instead of can vegetables. They hold more nutrient value than the can but if the can is all you have make sure you use the salt free vegetables. All can vegetables should be rinsed off to remove some of the sodium content.

6. **How long before I will notice a weight loss?**

As soon as thirty days. You will notice a loss on the scale as soon as three weeks. Some will notice a loss sooner but do not be deceived you are only losing water weight at first. The average weight lost is three pounds to five pounds a month. When the body is accepting the weight loss you will find your weight holding but it will start back to dropping so stick to the program, especially when losing so you can achieve success.

7. **Can men and boys use this diet as well as women and girls or do they need to make changes?**

Yes, this program has been tried out on both men and women and it is adjustable to both. Nothing need be changed but you might find that you will want to increase the broth and salad if you find you are still a little hungry. For the most part this program will stand just as it is the design of the program is for you to eat your way thin and this applies to both sexes. Children and teens can use this format they will find eating this way fun because they can pick and choose what they want and there is no wrong choice as long as you stay within the programs guidelines.

8. **Can you eat out on this program or do all of the meals have to be eaten at home?**

Yes, eating out on this program can be fun once you know what qualifies. You will need to take your measuring cups with you so that any extra food can be brought home for another meal. Sticking to the required amount of food per eating session is important. It allows the body a chance to accept the change you are now instituting. I often would ask the waitress to bring me a takeout container before I even got the meal so that I could prepare myself to put the extra away before I started eating. You will find that many people will ask why the cups and admire the effort you are taking to lose weight.

9. **Will I have to cook separate meals for my family members?**

No. You do not have to cook separate meals for your family. I found that my family ate what I ate at mealtime and they were surprise to find out how much they were overeating.

10. **Do you have to use Canola Oil and Olive Oil? Why not Vegetable oil?**

Yes, you have to use either Olive oil or Canola oil when cooking or making the salad dressing.

Olive oil is the oil of choice it only takes a little while to adjust to the change. Other oils leave you facing the question as to whether or not it is a transfat oil or not. I found that using the extra virgin and light Olive oil and Canola oil was just as easy as using the other. Olive oil gives a unique flavor to the food and it often times improved the taste of the dish.

11. **You recommend taking a tablespoon of olive oil in the morning. Can you explain why you do?**

   The tablespoon of olive oil in the morning upon rising helps with the body being kept regular. I found I didn't have a problem with constipation and the condition of your skin improves with its use. You might have to adjust to taking the oil you can improve the flavor by adding a little lemon juice or diet sweeter or by drinking a glass of juice right after digesting so as to take the taste out of your mouth. You can skip the oil in the morning I only suggest it you can use whatever you feel makes you comfortable with your digestion.

12. **Why do you suggest not weighing yourself during the first couple of months?**

   Weighing yourself when you first start the program is important because you need to know your start weight. I do not recommend you getting on the scale more than once a month. It is not necessary to weigh yourself you will find that it takes a lot of pressure off of you when you don't have to get up on that scale. I enjoyed weighing myself every three weeks and I would do it at the same time of day. I remember the first time I stepped on the scale after starting this program and how happy I was to see any weight loss. There is enough stress on you already in trying to keep to the program don't complicate it by adding the stress of weighing yourself everyday it's just not necessary.

13. **Why do you recommend buying a full length mirror?**

Most overweight people do not have a full length mirror in their home. I recommend you buy one so you will know exactly how you look from head to toe. I will never get over the shock I went through when the doctor took pictures of me both front and side views. I hadn't seen a side view of myself in over twenty years. I had no idea what I looked like and even worst was how it affected the way I felt about myself when I saw how I looked. I also recommend having someone take pictures of you front, back and side so you can have them to refer to after losing your desired weight. Don't be afraid of the mirror it's important to know what your body looks like and it will help you in reaching your goal. I put the picture of my behind on my refrigerator to motivate me into sticking to the program. I was shock to see what I looked like and every time I went to the fridge and saw the picture I often would turn around and go and do something else.

14. **Why do you recommend drinking water and liquids in general after the meal and not during it?**

I found that drinking water during the meal or liquids only confused the stomach into thinking you were full. I myself would take a few sips to rinse out my mouth but kept to drinking afterwards. You don't want to fill up on liquids instead of food. For one you will be hungry sooner if you do, liquids give you a false sense of fullness and when the liquid is digested you will find you are very hungry. The method of drinking afterwards is to help you when it comes to controlling your appetite. I recommend drinking liquids in between meals to help with the hunger feeling you often get when dieting.

15. **Why the large amount of fruit and vegetables in your program?**

Fruits and vegetables contain a great deal of water in them so I increase the amounts eaten during a setting. As with liquids you will feel full sooner and then feel hungry sooner once digested. The increase of fruits and vegetables help to stable out the body and helps you reach your goal easier. In this program everything is designed to help you reach your goal and help you maintain your goal weight once you reach it. Learn to mix your method of eating the fruits and vegetables up. If you are use to eating cooked vegetables try substituting raw vegetables instead. The same can be done with fruit this is to help you not to become bored with the process.

16. **You had Bariatric surgery done but don't recommend it, why?**

I was in danger of having a major heart attack at the time of my surgery. I was already losing weight with the program the surgery was to increase the loss quicker. I found the surgery to be extremely painful and there are dangers that you face with the surgery that add stress. Many people after having the surgery often gain the weight back because they haven't learned how to eat it off. I have found that for the most part anyone can follow the program without surgery and that it takes a little more time but the results are the same. I suggest that you try learning to eat it off and that way once you reach your goal weight you don't have to worry about learning how to maintain because you have learned it while you were taking it off. I have lost over 370 pounds and haven't had any problems in keeping it off because of how I learned to eat it off. Control was something which I had to learn and that is something most of the overweight people needed to learn. Surgery will only confuse the issue it will not help if you haven't learned how to properly eat.

There is no end to the Bariatric program you always have the fear of something going wrong so why add the stress unless you have to.

To the Bariatric team that worked on me and the inspiration they gave I give thanks. If surgery will help you obtain your goal and you choose it and commit to the lifestyle then I give my blessing but for myself I have found the lifestyle to be scary at times, especially the fact you have no stopping reality speaking. Make sure you are going to commit to the lifestyle and how you achieve your goal will be obtainable. This program was designed by a Bariatric patient. I had the surgery in 2006 after losing 175lbs. I had developed the program into practice and found it to work not just on myself but for others who concentrated on the program itself. Controlled nutrition is something that we all need, some may find they exist only with the knowledge of controlling and learning control is what will help them obtain success.

17. **Did you have problems dealing with your physical appearance after losing weight? How did your close friends and family react to your success?**

    When the weight started rapidly coming off I no longer had control of how I was eating and losing gradually. On the program WALKFREE teaches you learn to eat healthy. Regardless to who you are you have to practice control in order to exist. When you learn to control your eating and how to maintain a healthy lifestyle on a simple budget your goals seem more achievable.

What bothered me most was the fact that my family saw the surgery and not the effort put forth to get the weight off. I learned how to eat my way to the body I wanted. I also learned how to exercise and incorporate it into my life daily. I believe my success came from wanting to live a healthier lifestyle and wanting to be here for my children and grandchildren.

18. **What kept you focused while you were dieting when it came to your outward appearance? How were you able to keep up with the wardrobe when losing weight?**

My family and friends but mostly it was my grandchildren. They had no doubt I could lose the weight and they were right. Children accept you just as you are but more important they aren't afraid to point out the flaws. My grandson at two would walk up to my thigh and point to the extra skin. I would be so embarrassed but he was a child so what could I do but accept his innocence. How I kept up with wardrobe was by shopping at resale shops and flea markets. I found I could find cloths easier once I was losing weight.

19. **Did you need surgery afterwards to remove the excess skin?**

> Yes. I had to have 17 pounds of excess skin removed from my stomach but I have not been able to afford to have my arms or my thighs done. My breasts need to be done also but I doubt if I will ever be able to afford to have it done. The state I was in paid for the stomach surgery but they refused my thigh and arms. I looked like the elephants had loaned me their ears at first. I exercise regularly and it is my hopes to one day tighten my loose skin.

20. **Did your health improve after the weight loss?**

> Yes, my overall health improved for instance I had high blood pressure, but now it's normal. I suffer from asthma and nothing has changed there but I had a problem with arthritis and still have a problem with the discomfort. I will admit that it is not as painful now as it was before I loss the weight. You see in general my health did improve but I make this point sternly losing weight is not a miracle cure. You will still face problems once you lose the weight and if you go into this unrealistically you will cause yourself to build up false hope and it will halter your success.

Tips, Tips and more Tips
(Everything helps on your road to success)

When I first started losing weight I had no one to help me with the questions I had running through my mind. I cannot tell you how stressful it was trying to sort my way through the maze of weight programs and diets. I thought I was going to pull my hair out one night trying to figure out what to eat for dinner. I think it was that night that I realized I had to come up with a better way for me to succeed. Now I am not a miracle worker the following tips are things which I tried and worked and I pass them on to you so that you too might have success. So the first place we will begin is with drinking water. I know that water is important but another important fact is that water is in everything that we consume. I cannot stress it enough that you will need to drink at least 6-8 glasses of water in order for your body to eliminate the waste material properly.

You can count water intake in fruit and vegetables as well as in the diet sodas, teas and coffee you consume.

Remember that water is necessary so find a way to make it enjoyable. I tried putting fresh basil in water in a pitcher and filling it with ice and lemon slices. The water takes on a different flavor and the change is refreshing. Another favorite of mind was taking citrus fruit and slicing it thin and putting the slices in water. Fresh berries are great for crushing and putting in water for the flavor you will find not all fruit makes a good addition to the water but most of them can add a smile to your face.

I tried to steer clear of the diet sodas mainly because of the sodium which is inside. I found that if you steer clear of items that have high sodium you will find you get some control on swelling especially in the feet.

I enjoyed finding things to eat that helped eliminate water in the body naturally. Some vegetables that help naturally relieve the body of water is celery, mushrooms, green peppers just to mention a few. I would make myself a tray of water I call the water veggies and eat them every day. I believe in doing it naturally if at all possible so I found myself going into the health stores and doing a lot of researching. For one thing I found out that a lot of over the counter drugs and health products conflict with the medicines I was taking. Make sure you check with your doctor to find out whether or not something is safe for you to take.

I found that for the most part most diets are the same in what they tell you are necessary for you to lose weight. Now where they differ in how you go about it, I found that I began to lose weight once I took my find off weight and put it on food. I began to study food and found that if I ate six meals instead of three that I didn't feel like I was cheating myself out of something. I recommend that you try eating every three hours like I did and see how it works for you. I would break my meals down to three main and three small meals. The main meals would contain the meat and the smaller meals the emphasis was on fruits and vegetables. I began to have fun making up the smaller meals and finding ways to create things to eat that I hadn't had before. I would make cheese and cracker platters which would contain my fruit and numerous vegetables.

One of my favorite things to make is a tortilla filled with sautéed vegetables. I also liked taking refried beans and making what I call a bean pizza. You take a tortilla and cover it with refried beans, sprinkle a little cheese on it and top it with a few slice olives. Heat on stove top just until the cheese is melted and slice in half. It's a great way to eat protein and its rather filling and very low cal.

A good trick with eggs is to use one whole egg with two egg whites when making omelets. I got my family eating vegetable omelets by sautéing the vegetables first. A great omelet which even children likes is in 2 tablespoon of light olive oil salute a small onion which has been sliced thin, 4 mushrooms sliced thin, ½ carrot grated, ¼ green pepper until soften. Beat the egg and whites and season with 2 tablespoons of fresh chopped basil. Pour the eggs on top and sprinkle with garlic powder and onion powder and a little chili powder. You can use a vegetable spray instead of oil when cooking the omelet let it cook slow flip when golden. I sprinkle the top with a little cheese.

I found that you can make a olive and onion topping and let it sit in the refrigerator for a few minutes before serving with crackers. Take 20 black olives chopped fine, and ½ small red onions diced, 1 small diced tomato, ¼ teaspoon of basil, 1teaspoon minced garlic mix together and store in container. Serve with crackers or toasted pitas.

I found making my own pita chips to be a fun adventure for the whole family. I take tortilla chips and cut them in half and quarter them. I then spray them down with olive oil and then season them with various herbs. I like using chili powder and cayenne pepper along with a little black pepper for the spicy chip. I have made onion flavor and garlic chips. Bake them in a 400 degree oven until golden about ten minutes. I like making my own dip I use onion power and parsley, basil, garlic powder and a little diet sweetener to 1 cup of sour cream. To give it a little substance I add 3 tablespoons of plain yogurt. I don't use the onion packets because they contain too much salt I found it easier to just make my own creations. I have even taken yogurt and added crushed fruit and blended it together with a little diet sweetener. It makes a great dip for fruit as well as crackers.

When it comes to losing weight you have to use your imagination. I found that if it didn't look good or smell good I didn't want it. I had to make myself get use to eating the vegetables and fruit. I learned to create dishes that I liked which were loaded with calories and make them diet friendly.

I love banana pudding so I learned to make one with graham crackers and low calorie pudding mix. The key is to use all sugar free items and to layer the pudding with bananas and to go light on the crackers. I would add banana flavor to the pudding to boost the flavor along.

I learned to make cobbler by using sugar free fruit and sweetener and for the crust I would use puff pastry which I had rolled out extremely thin. I put the emphasis on the fruit and would always layer the fruit the top with the puff pastry and sprinkle with a little diet sweetener I found Splenda is great for cooking and doesn't leave an after taste in the mouth.

I love ice cream and found that I liked making my own better than the one in the store. I like using peaches, bananas when making ice cream they seem to give the most flavors. Try leaving chunks of fruit in the ice cream and mixing a couple of cherries in for color. Remember that the appearance of the food is what satisfies the mind.

Many people laughed when I started carrying my measuring cups around but I had the last laugh. I used the cups to help me get control of my eating. I was overeating and didn't know it. With the cups you learn to see just what a cup of a certain item is. I didn't realize that most of the food I was consuming was too much. Once you start measuring your food you soon will be able to recognize what a cup of something looks like and there is a feeling of power in knowing I have the control of the situation. I look at all the people who are buying into these programs which send you the food already packaged. All they are teaching you is how to monitor your food so I decided to take charge and create my own dishes.

Remember that the palm of your hand holds the size of meat you can consume. If you stick to the palm and no thicker than your thumb you will find that you pretty much can monitor your meat and keep the control needed. I don't recommend you eating more than 6-8 ounces of meat a day. I stress the importance of you monitoring the beef you consume. Beef takes three days to leave the body so if you eat it more than once you are defeating your goal. I enjoy having a burger or steak but I don't want to carry it all week around with me.

I didn't lose 370 pounds overnight it took me months of trying before I got the right process. I want you to try different things but to keep in mind that you can't achieve your goal of losing weight if you don't monitor yourself. You have to eat to lose weight and you have to eat healthy in order to lose and achieve your goal. The one good thing about learning to eat healthy is that I didn't have to teach myself anything new when it came to maintaining. I am eating the same food which I ate to get thin and that is what makes the difference. If you don't take time to learn to cook and eat healthy you are defeating yourself before you start.

Learning how to take the fat out of food and how to give food flavor takes a little time. You first have to adjust to the change yourself so doesn't worry when you falter simply continue on. I didn't have failure I had trial and error. If something didn't come out right I tried something else. You learn what vegetables your body can adjust to and what ones you have to stay away from. Just about any vegetable can be cooked and many can be used in the place of meat. I found that Portabella mushroom are expensive but if you replace meat with them they balance out in a budget. Mushrooms are meaty and when you par them with onions and green peppers and salute them until tender they make a very good sandwich. I have eaten them as sandwiches and subs as well as in pitas.

My oil of choice is olive oil and I live by it. I like to use various blends when cooking. I like adding lemon peel and orange peel to the olive oil for salads. I like putting a little pepper flakes and garlic for a little spice. You can try experimenting and creating your own family favorites. I also recommend olive oil as a way of keeping the body regular. I take a tablespoon every morning you can put a little mustard and diet sweetener in it for flavor. A little olive oil goes a long way and it's healthy. Try sampling different olive oil and finding the one which suits your taste buds.

My family likes fried foods so I learned to bake a pretty good fake out chicken in the oven. I use a mixture of cornmeal and flour which gives the meat a little crunch. I have even crushed up cornflakes and rice kipsies and used them as a coating. The main thing is to add herbs to the coating. A good crunchy coating for chicken is ½ cup flour, ¼ cup of corn meal, 1 teaspoon pepper,

1 teaspoon garlic powder, 1 teaspoon onion powder, 1 teaspoon paprika, ¼ teaspoon poultry seasoning, ½ cup cornflakes crushed fine. Mix well in bowl. Season the chicken with garlic powder and onion powder and black pepper dip in egg whites and then into the coating mix. Place on a baking sheet which has been sprayed with non stick spray. Spray the chicken down with a light coating of vegetable spray and cook in a preheated oven 400 degrees until done. I like coating the chicken and letting it sit about fifteen minutes before cooking so the meat has a chance to pick up the flavor of the herbs. Did you notice that I used a lot of herbs and spices? I started experimenting with the herbs after watching a television cooking show. Personally I favor Basil its multi use helps even more. It's important as with anything you do to learn the base point.

When it comes to learning how to eat healthy the first step is learning how to pacify your taste buds. To achieve that you must first go through a period of trial and error. Once you know what you like then you can learn how to process it in your daily living.

The problem I found with most diets is the fact that they more or less want you to stick to what they say to eat. I found that I couldn't afford most of the things they had on the list of items to eat. I began to research what foods are good in the body and easy when it comes to being eliminated from the body. I found that there was really no bad food but that some foods you had to monitor as to how much and when we ate them. Beef for instance takes three days to leave the body but if you eat less at a serving you have more control. I found that using a sirloin which has very little fat to be a better choice than ground round. You have to at all times consider the fat which is in the food and also the fat you are putting into the food. Everyone needs a little fat in their system so to think you can live without fat is fruitless. What you have to do is learn to put the right amount of fat into your system and how to remove the excess fat from the food. It takes time also to readjust to the taste of the fat missing from the food. You will be surprise at how we have accustomed our taste buds to accept grease as normal. I remember when I made my first burger without all the fat I felt it was rather dry. It wasn't that it was dry I was missing all the grease dripping so I associated it with dryness. I now enjoy eating a burger and don't miss the fat at all which has been taken out. The same thing can be said about fried foods. You miss the greasy taste that over the years you related to as normal. Once you try baking the chicken with a little crunch you'll notice that it's not half as bad as you thought it would be. In fact most people feel it's a pretty good substitute for the fried chicken.

These series of tips are written in the hopes to help you along the journey you are partaking. I realized when I started that I would have probably not had so many setbacks if I had know some of the things mention in this chapter. None of the tips are meant to be full proof what works for one person might not work for another. But in general these tips have been found helpful by everyone. As with anything you have to stick to it in order to see the results you want. You can't expect to see a miracle happen overnight, after all you didn't put the weight on overnight it took years of eating.

Remember to give yourself a little time and to focus on treating yourself special whether you lose one pound or ten. I tried everything I could to stick to the diet plans which the doctors gave me but I found it hard and most times impossible. For one I had a hard time getting all of the food which they wanted me to consume. I had no idea what to replace the expensive meats with and so it caused me to resort back to my old eating habits after a while. I really wanted to succeed but I felt like I was already defeated if I couldn't stick to the program prescribed. So I started researching food in regards to price and how to use it in cooking and fitting all of it into my budget. One of the first things I learned was that more than a meat being able to fix in my budget it had to come across with the flavor needed for me to accept it. That's where the trial and error came in and I learned a lot about what meats work well in dieting and which ones need to me monitored. An important fact to remember is that if it doesn't taste good to you or isn't appealing drop it from your menu.

Sure you could have it shipped to you already packed but wouldn't it be fun to plan your own meals with things you truly can enjoy? The problem with buying the food and having it delivered is when you no longer can afford to have it done. It's then you realize that you should have learned how to prepare the meals. I feel it was better for me to learn as I lost that way I didn't have to worry about the future.

One of the most asked questions since I have lost the weight is wasn't it easy since I had Bariatric Surgery done. I cannot stress this enough that it doesn't matter if you have the surgery or not. If you don't know how to eat healthy and cook healthy the weight that you lose will soon creep back up on you. Weight loss comes from what you learn about control and how you apply it to your life. If you don't know control you can't control your weight and gaining is the only option. I wanted to lose and keep it off and surgery or not had to learn healthy living. I found that healthy living is what leads to a longer life and when I started learning portion control and how to cook my food so that it was healthy and full of flavor my weight simply came off. I owe my life to the doctor who performed the surgery on me. He saved my life but it was me alone which learned how to eat and live a more healthy life. Surgery did do one thing for me it caused me to develop excessive skin pockets. I had a problem keeping the skin tight with such rapid weight loss and the fact I was so large made it difficult to exercise. I learned the importance of exercise in a weight loss program. Exercise is what helps tones the skin so that as you lose the skin tightens along with you and you don't wind up with elephant ears flapping in the wind. Once again I stress that these are only tips but you have to put them into action and make them work for you.

In the course of a day I am often asked over and over again did I feel like cheating or stopping the diet? On any diet a person can get the feeling that they want to have something which is not on the program they are following. The important fact to remember is that we are human and that we are subject to have feeling such as these. I found that it was easier for me to simply go ahead and eat what was weighing so heavy on my mind. Better that you eat a little of something which you think you want than to have it haunting your mind like a weight. I don't suggest you overeat but a small amount of what you think you want may be all you need to pacify your desire.

I remember having a taste for fried chicken and French fries. I had the feeling I had to have the chicken all day and I was getting stressed thinking about it. I was on my way to pick up some fruit from the market and right next door there was a Kentucky Fried Chicken. I found myself pulling into the lot and going inside and ordering. I usually would have ordered three or four pieces of chicken but instead I simply ordered one piece. I went and got back into my car and sat there and ate the one piece of chicken out of the view of everyone in my family. It was one thing I wanted to cheat but another that I wanted to get everyone involved talking about it. Family and friends and be cruel when it comes to you cheating. Especially if you have been doing good following your program but what was worse having the thought drive you crazy or you simply eating a piece of chicken? I ate the one piece and was satisfied and didn't want more, in fact I didn't want fried chicken again while I was trying to reach my goal weight. This taught me something that if you satisfy a desire which is overriding you that you gain a form of control over the situation. I didn't think of it as cheating but as moving forward on handling control over my food. I was proud that I didn't overeat the chicken and

I didn't mention it to my family. What would they have added a pat on the back?

Another major question was about exercising and when you should start a regular routine. I wish I had started working out sooner but I wasn't able to move very well when I first started the program. I was so big that I had difficulty standing as well as sitting down. I had to wait until I had lost some weight before I could start a regular workout program. I really want to stress now that it is important to work out from the beginning so that you can help firm the muscles. By waiting so long I only created other problems for myself. I had Bariatric Surgery done because of the problems I was having with my health. I had lost over one and seventy pounds before the surgery and had started exercising regularly. Once the healing process of the surgery was over the weight began to drop off at such an increase rate that my skin which was at the time tight became very loose. In fact I was unable to tighten the skin and keep up with the weight loss. This was disturbing for me I am a woman who regardless of my size always was rather vain. I didn't want my skin to look so wrinkled and when I found out the state was not going to pay for anymore surgeries I became concern. I believe if I had been working out right along it still would not have made that much of a difference since the weight was coming off faster that I could tone it. In my health club I stress the importance of doing sit down exercising or what is known as couch potatoes workouts. These workouts give the overweight person an advantage they allow you to work out the muscle while sitting down.

This is not a cure for excessive skin but it will help in forming the new muscle and the more you workout the better the muscle tone. Until you can add another workout program to your daily routine stick to the couch potato one better to be working out than not doing any form of workout program at all.

Did I listen to other workout coaches or did you still to just one? I listen and learned a little from everyone I watched or studied. There is no full proof way to tone the body or get the weight off. Each instructor has their own method which they think will work when it come to taking the weight off. For the most part the program does work but not one everyone I stuck to a diet plan and worked out every day but I gained weight instead of losing. For one I was not eating right I was taking medicine which didn't react well with the food I was taking. You have to be careful to watch out for your health when you are trying to lose weight. The same is true for working out you have to make sure you aren't hurting yourself by doing it wrong or by overworking the muscle. I couldn't move my lower body very well so I spent a great deal of time overworking out the upper body. This left me sore and soon I began to slow down because of the discomfort.

Most of us can't afford a personal weight trainer and if we could would we follow everything they said? I learned to do a little everyday was the key and I started using the muscles I could control. What happen was I begun to look better my upper body was firming but my lower wasn't. I learned through this that it is important to work the whole body even at a slow rate so that the overall effect of the program can be felt. Beauty must be worked on and it takes time. Like lipstick you might have to wipe it off and start all over again to get the effect you want.

Patience is something which you must have if you are going on any diet program. Patience to remember that you didn't get this way over night and it will not disappear overnight. You will have to work at learning how to eat correctly and also on how to tighten the skin. It is foolish to think that you will not have to do any form of exercising and we have the best form of workout available to us.

Walking. I started walking with a walker and could barely get around at first but each day I attempted to walk a little further until I was actually walking a regular routine. I would go out for fifteen minutes a day and try to walk until I could walk. I suggest that you attempt the same thing try walking to the corner or just to a chair and back. The effort is what is important not the amount of time put into it. You have to walk correctly so not to hurt yourself, I found it funny that I had to learn to walk correctly so that I didn't hurt my back more. The more I walked the less pain I began to feel and that was the plus side.

Many people thought I was sick because of the rapid weight loss. They were used to seeing me overweight and not trying to do anything about it. When they saw me suddenly working out and sticking to the program they were concern I was over doing it. Strange no one thinks you're overdoing it when you are stuffing yourself or not working out. I believe people have good intentions such as my friends and family they just didn't know that they were adding to the problem when they weren't supporting the effort. Any effort you put forth to change your situation should be accepted as right and good. My walking was limited but it was helping and with each day I got better and soon I learned to tone out the voices of people and focus on what I was attempting to do.

Over the three years it took me to lose the weight I rearranged numerous menus. Many I took things out that I didn't like and others I added things on that I did. I enclosed at the end of this book some of the recipes that I found to be enjoyable while I was losing, and even now that I am maintaining my weight. I didn't have to relearn any special program once I reached my goal weight mainly because the program I was on was one of accuracy. I learned to properly eat the correct amount of an item. For instance I use to eat fruit everyday but I didn't eat enough fruit. Now I make a point in consuming my fruit right along with my meal but I also have it as a treat during the day. The same can be said about vegetables we have to learn to make eating the correct amount more important than anything.

Overeating causes more problems and it's harder to stop if you don't know you're doing wrong. I didn't know eating two apples could be changed to eating a apple with a little peanut butter. The peanut butter is added protein and helps to cut the appetite. So I could have a little something sweet as well as give the muscle a little treat also. When losing you has to learn to put everything together to work for the outcome you want. If you don't know what is the proper amount then you are subject to overeat whether you want to or not.

Nearly everything you eat can be substituted for something healthy. I found that even when I craved Ice cream that I could substitute frozen yogurt with fruit and that it worked. Sure I had to be willing to accept the yogurt as the substitute in order for the idea to work. I learned that with anything you have to be willing to try something new to replace the old. If you are a fried chicken buff you will have to readjust to eating oven fried chicken. Sure it will take a moment or two to accept it but once you have accepted it you will only be helping yourself to reach your goal. To lose weight something has to be given up!

I was never a water buff I drank water only when I had to. So the fact I had to drink eight or more glasses was defeating at first. I learned to flavor my water and to adjust to drinking low calorie or sugar free drinks. Keeping in mind that it is better for you to make your own because that way you control the sodium content. Most sugar free sodas have high sodium content and salt is dangerous if not monitored. Salt is in everything from can goods to water so be careful and remember to watch what you are putting into your body. Too much salt will cause swelling and that is something you don't want to happen. I walked on swollen feet for years and the pain was always unbearable. I welcome learning how to control the salt and was overjoyed when the swelling began to go down. I can't tell you how happy I am to be able to walk now and not feel that knifing pain in my feet.

I'm often asked what do I use on my skin it looks so healthy. I must admit that I don't use any special items at all. I do standby moisturizing the skin for it is only way to keep the elasticity and that is needed when losing weight. You can't tighten skin that doesn't have elasticity and dry skin jut doesn't look or react well to dieting. So from the first day moisturize your skin and try experimenting with different creams until you find the one that is best for your skin. I had to try numerous one and finally had to mix up my own lotion from three that were on the market. Each one gave my skin a little of what it needed but all three together gave my skin the added boost needed to keep the moisture in.

Don't overeat the sugar free treats! I did at first I thought because it was sugar free that it wouldn't hurt me and it was just the opposite. I was eating too much and it was causing me to visit the bathroom regularly. Diet sweetener can cause you to have the runs if you eat too much of it so be careful not to. You have to consider what you are drinking as well as what you are eating and monitor all of it. Nothing is put to chance when dieting you have to be a expert at controlling any situation when it comes to what goes into your body. Most overweight people got that way because they didn't watch what they put inside their bodies. They ate what they wanted and the price for that was added weight. You can still eat what you want but you practice control and it's that control that allows the body to adjust to change and with change comes hope of success. It's all tied in together and for it to work well you have to apply all that you learn to memory.

One of the reasons many diets fail is because you haven't learned to put control into your system.

Control, control and more control that is what it takes to reach your goal weight. I found it fun to try to put my memory to the test and see if I could remember just how much of an item I could eat. I didn't want learning control over food to stop me from succeeding. I didn't get it right away it took months of practice before I finally got it. Even then I find myself overeating an item so don't feel bad if it happens to you. Just start all over again and with time you too will be losing with a smile. From childhood we are taught to overeat and not pay attention to what we are consuming. We love to say what is bad for the body but not what is good. Control over food comes from learning and that is a proven fact. If you are not willing to learn control chances are you won't reach your goal so buckle up and learn to start controlling your intake of food.

Don't be surprised if you question the amounts I did but as time went by I began to see that I was getting full on the controlled amount and didn't need the extra as I thought.

These tips won't help unless you're willing to apply them to your life. You have everything to look forward to as the weight begins to come off and you begin to put what you learn into action. It takes time for the mind to accept the change but once it does things begin to move quickly. I hope that something I mention in this chapter will help you as you work your way toward your goal of success. Again I advise you to check with your doctor before putting this program into action. I am not a doctor only a person who has lost over 370 pounds and kept records which I now pass on to you. I know that it is hard to start a diet when you weigh so much. I hope that this book will encourage the reader to want to start the program and then succeed at their goal of reaching their goal weight.

Learning Can Be Fun!

"You can't teach a old dog new tricks!" I still remember the lady who said that to me and I say to her again "You Can Too!!!" I was thirty eight when my weight got totally out of control and began affecting my health. I was up until that time what I considered to be an okay person. I considered myself to be normal or average. I had lived a rather wild and racy lifestyle and my weight went along with the life I was leading. MY catering business was growing and I was in the right field I loved cooking and even more I loved eating. You have to know yourself and I knew one thing I loved to cook food and even more I loved to eat it. So when my weight became a problem I overlooked it and used my field to hide behind. It was easier for me to say that I had to taste my food as an excuse for eating. I simply was putting on more and more pounds and the truth of the matter is if I hadn't had the mild stroke I probably would not have changed my attitude or life. I was dying but it didn't matter I was not going to give up my food. It was the only luxury that I had that life hadn't taken away.

Are you feeling something like that? I had to see I had a problem in order to get help and help myself. Most of the overweight people in the world would change if it could happen overnight. But that is a dream so most people simply hide behind the truth. I spent years telling people I had a thyroid problem whether than admit I had a problem with controlling myself. I thought I had self control but the truth was I didn't when it came to eating. I would eat for all the wrong reasons I celebrated good things with eating as well as the depression with eating. I spent most of my time in the kitchen anyway so food was easy to turn to. I was beginning to cook healthy simply because of the times changing in the food world. People were asking for healthier menus to pick from and I was adjusting to my financial pocket not my taste buds. I had a business which called for me to be around food but that was not good in my case. I had been hiding behind the food for years when my marriage went bad I ate, when my health began to fail I ate, when problems happen with the children I ate, do you see a familiar pattern. I was eating and getting bigger and all of it was getting out of control. When I had to lose fifty pounds I would say I would work on it next month. But as the pounds mounted I soon had to lose an hundred then two hundred and soon I wasn't thinking about losing weight anymore.

For one I didn't understand why if I was cooking healthier why wasn't I losing weight? I was eating the food I was cooking and the diet books swore I should lose ten pounds why I didn't? I was overeating and instead of losing I was gaining. The same food which was meant to make me healthy was killing me only because I lacked control. I found that control when it comes to dieting has to be learned. It is something that the mind, heart and soul have to accept in order for it to work. I wanted to lose but I didn't want to feel cheated when it came to eating. I would try hard to follow the diets given to me by doctors but they weren't working because I wasn't putting them into effect. I had a problem I was not accepting it so even though the mind was ready the heart wasn't. For any diet program to work you first have to admit you have a problem. Be willing to change the problem by learning how to readjust. Be willing to work at changing this seems simple at first but it isn't. Change is something that the heart has to accept and then the mind before the stomach will okay it. I had a lot of heart but when it came to will power and self control I had a lot to learn. I had pride also I didn't want to admit I didn't have self control over my eating. I would often tell people that I ate like a bird but I didn't say what size bird!

Doctors give you diets to follow they don't tell you how to come up with the food to eat on those diets. The average person is on a very tight budget and just can't afford to diet unless they learn some tips to help them on the change. I had to learn not only how to shop but how to buy better in order for it to last longer. Strange statement isn't it I had to learn to buy better? I use to buy pork and I still do but instead of the pork butt I buy the pork loin. I cook it slowly and slice it thinly and place it into storage bags in 3ounce servings. I can reenter this meat into my diet in numerous ways and now I no longer have to worry about the grease, I eliminated the problem. Not all meat can be done like this but I take advantage of the ones that can. Learning to put my meat in 3ounce portions; helped when it came to recognizing correct proportion and gaining control on your eating. I soon began to recognize I had too much meat on my plate when I was out at restaurants or my friends and families. I began to carry mini storage bags and put my extra away for another meal. I started taking the bones out of the meat and weighing just meat so that I could learn what the meat looked like when its portion was accurate. I had been overeating and didn't know it and was surprise to find out I was satisfied on the three ounces. I had brainwashed myself into believing that too much was enough. It took several months of practice before I accepted that the right portion was sufficient and I was content.

I had to learn how to make it appealing to the sight as well as the tongue. I can't stand for food to look bland and taste like cardboard. I believe in flavor and it has to look good in order for me to enjoy it. I learned to par my meats with colorful vegetables that brought out their flavor even more. Each meal became a diner's feast and I would sit down to enjoy the fruits of my labor. When I took the time to measure everything at first it seemed long and dragged out but as time went by I found it fun to see just how much each item would fill my plate. On days that I was extremely hungry I would use fruits and vegetables which looked like I had a lot. For example, when I am extremely hungry I will eat grapes, crushed fruit in diet Jell-O, which I cut into squares. I enjoy peanuts and sliced olives I make myself a plate of fruits and vegetables and put a dip in the middle. I nibble on a legal snack all day and the desire to cheat is lessen. I stick close to the proper amounts so that I overeat. When I first started I had to measure or weigh but now I know the amounts in my head and I simply fix my plate accordingly.

Making sure you make the food appealing is important if you want to stay focus and reach your goal. If you tire of eating one thing; change, and even try cooking it another way. Variety is what makes any diet program a success. I learned to eat a variety of foods and took time to research for other foods with the same nutrient value. Mixing fruit with yogurt and Jell-O changes the appearance. I even found a way to make a frozen treat with my fruits and all of it helped in aiding my getting control of my eating. By consuming protein with nearly every meal I found my hunger level to be lower. Sardines and five crackers can get you through to your next meal; you don't like sardines well substitute mushrooms or maybe mussels. You don't need a bowl full only a few ounces to cut the hunger. I don't deny myself food I simply treat myself to the correct portion and enjoy it.

Don't fall prey to the tricks which our minds play on us when we are trying to institute a change. For instance I knew I had to start monitoring the amounts of my food but I kept making excuses for not doing it. I kept saying I would start tomorrow but when tomorrow came I had another excuse. I found that if you are going to start something there is no time like the present. I began measuring with a frown but it soon became a smile when the pounds started coming off. The best things in life don't come easy" I heard that statement often enough. The truth of the matter is that the best thing I could have done was learn portion control. I don't think I could express how happy or how much safer I felt on the program once I learned my cup and half cup measurements.

Once I was able to recognize three ounces and replace my overeating with control eating. As the weight began to drop off my self esteem rose and I found that others who had been teasing me were now paying attention to what I was doing. We need a little fat to lubricate these old bones of ours. That's why I recommend you take a tablespoon of olive oil a day. Just like an apple it's good for what ails you. Olive oil is a proven miracle and something that can be adapted to most menus. I found that olive oil in some dishes gave it the boost of flavor it needed. Before saying it won't work for you try creating flavors that you like? I like sweet and spicy oils but when it comes to cooking I like the plain light oils. I try to substitute olive oil for any oil that calls for a vegetable oil or fat. I don't think the difference is noticeable and for the most part neither is the flavor.

Doctors like to stick to proven facts but all facts came from someone trying them out first. I didn't like the fact no one gave me extra money to buy groceries yet expected me to follow their program. I didn't know I could substitute meats and get the same effect. I had to learn how to replace a meat with a meat of equal value when it came to taste, and how it cooked on the plate. If something doesn't appeal to your sense of taste then you will not eat it. Canned meat is a better value at times but it holds more sodium. I learned to substitute it but not add salt or products which contain high salt levels. Canned chicken if boiled first makes a good broth for cooking and once cooled can be used in most menus the same as fresh meat; it just takes a little practice.

Fresh fruits and vegetables are a little more costly but the flavor and taste can't be matched. I found buying fruit and vegetables which are in season to be a better buy. The fun comes in learning how to if them differently and more creatively. Healthy eating is fun because you learn not only to readjust you're eating but are open to accepting new flavors and ideas. I like fresh green beans and frozen ones to the can. I like the crunch you get from the fresh that you lose in the can. When it comes to pineapple and pears I like the can because you can't find a better taste than that of the can to me. Your taste might be different so try it and if you like it the other way around then go with what makes you happy. Remember I believe food is to be enjoyed and that applies to whether you are on a diet or not.

No one can design a meal plan for you better than yourself. I had all kinds of help but it wasn't until I started learning how to plan my own meals that I truly began to understand what healthy eating was all about. As with any diet program you need to know the basics to help it work.

Even controls meals have a program they want you to follow so the plan can work better. I found that it wasn't wise to start something I know I couldn't keep up especially when it came to me losing weight. I had to have a way of keeping fruit and vegetables in my life and it had to be on my budget. One of the things I learned is how to rotate food choices. If you start the day with a canned fruit then change it to a fresh fruit during the day. Don't eat the same thing over and over without changing it a little bit. The change is what you will learn helps you stay focus. When we can apply variety we feel we have control. Now no one has been able to understand why for some that control is so hard to establish. For some the change comes easy to follow and set in motion. That is the same as with most things in life we have the power to control ourselves with time. You want to stop smoking you can once you learn some tricks that help you gain control. Well food is the same way you can learn some tricks to help you stay focus. If you like munching then you have to find out what vegetables and fruit are good for you to munch on. You can't expect to quit munching just because you are on a diet or control food menu.

I know a friend who was on one of the controlled food programs. She had been paying all that money to eat and hadn't learned how to do it if her circumstances changed. When she became laid off she found she couldn't afford the food so she had to break down and ask me for some of my menus. I have taken menu from hundreds of books over the years and made them cost efficient or taste worthy. She didn't know how to stay on the diet without the prepackaged food. I always say that if you learn on the package it will so box you out. The time she had to spend relearning how to eat could have been avoided if she had simply learned how to if the meals herself from the beginning.

Short cuts can be dangerous if not properly thought out. If you are going to use the prepackage program make sure you take time to learn to do it without the help of the package. The same can be said about surgery and its results. Yes, you will lose weight with the surgery but if you don't learn to properly eat. You will get to your goal weight but then find yourself gaining weight back. You have to know what foods to eat and the proper amount in order for the plan to work. If you learn how to cook the foods you like properly and the proper portion needed for consuming you can't help but maintain your goal.

You don't need thousands of dollars to teach you self control just a measuring cup or two will do it. Once again I tell you that none of it will work unless you are willing to take the time to learn how to do it. Can a old dog learn new tricks? Sure but it might take a little time for him to digest it and accept it.

Something I had to learn was how to dress to make myself feel better as well and look better. I had been use to hiding the fat under my clothes I was use to squeezing myself into some pair of stretch pants thinking it was making me look thinner. The truth of the matter I looked fatter once I squeezed my body into those pants and my breathing became a major issue. I would usually wind up using my inhaler because I was suddenly short of breath. I was choking myself out in the effort to look thinner. Have you done the same? Did it work? or did you too find yourself struggling to get out of the pants just so you could breathe?

I remember once that I had to rush into the kitchen and cut the stretch pants off of me so I could breathe. I was smothering myself all because I wanted to look thinner. I learned from that to wear clothes that had room to breathe. I didn't have to look like I had a tent on but I surely didn't have to wear something so tight I couldn't allow myself to breathe in them. No one overweight can brag about never trying to make them a little more beautiful. I remember one evening I became depress because the gown which I had been wearing for years had become destroyed in the washing machine. I put in a gown and pulled out sheds of material. When I saw the gown shredded I started crying and I couldn't figure out why for the longest. I couldn't understand why the gown being destroyed had caused such effect on me. The thing was I didn't go out in the public that much shopping and the gown was the only one I had. It meant me going out and buying a new one and I dreaded the idea. When I finally got up the nerve to go out shopping I was even more upset at the selection I had to choose from. Big women like looking good in bed people! I think the fashion world has improved in some ways but in other issues they have remained the same. No overweight woman or man looks good in shorts and tight shirts. We can cover up all we want but nothing will change the appearance of your body other than CHANGE!

I switched to jogging pants when it came to working out and found a nice pair of stretch pants which could be dressed up. This allowed me a change in my appearance. If you wear the same thing to church that you work out in you will not have a reason to change your appearance for the better. I went out and finally found a gown which looked pretty enough for me to buy. I learned that something as simple as a gown could defeat you if you don't have a handle on it. I didn't just come into control it came to me with practice.

I liked smelling good when I was big and still do not that I have reached my goal weight. I still like enjoying an evening snack upon retiring before I go to bed. I often drink a glass of skim milk and enjoy a sugar free cookie before retiring. I feel like I am giving myself a treat when I do so and it helps that I've learned to change that snack to yogurt and cookies or even fresh fruit. I like consuming calcium before I go to sleep at night you might not but might enjoy a cup of tea instead with a couple of cheese and crackers. Snacks can be made to be acceptable and legal it only means you have to learn how to substitute the right things on your menu.

Are you a sleep eater? Do you reach over to the nightstand and pick up a piece of candy or something else and put in your mouth when you wake up during the night? I found I was munching in my sleep so I started leaving healthy snacks around my bed. I notice a change in my weight the first month I hadn't realize how much I was overeating by my sleep munching. I was always telling people that I didn't eat a big meal and that was true because I usually ate while I was cooking. I would eat a piece of chicken to see it I had it flavored right. Or try a plate of greens to see I had enough pepper in them. Get the point? I was overeating with a blessing from myself. I didn't have room to put a full meal into my stomach after I had cooked a meal. Learning to stop eating was something which I had to practice. I didn't learn it easily I had problems in learning to not eat the whole piece of chicken and trusting my judgment that I had flavored the dish right. You can always taste the final product that's the good thing about using fresh or dried herbs it doesn't take long for the flavor to set into the food.

Replacing salt with flavor takes practice. You will find the world of spices opens many doors to changing a rather ordinary meal. I purchased a book on spices since I didn't know that much and wanted to learn more. It was an investment that I still use even today in my cooking. I also purchase a book on some of the things that I was studying like diabetes, cancer, stroke or heart problems I wanted to know how to eat healthy on all aspects of life. I didn't want to suffer another stroke so I practice heart healthy meals right along with my regular meals. I learned that it takes a little bit of everything to make the stew taste just right. It takes a little bit of learning a little of everything when it comes to reaching your goal weight. If you find you really miss the salt you can use a salt substitute but be careful for too much of this substitute will cause the same problems for you as regular salt.

No one person is the same so the weight comes off each of us differently. I found that if you follow this program that no matter whether you are a child or an adult that you can reach your goal weight. You have to make the change and it takes time to develop and remember the rules that will help you reach your goal. Nothing will change if you don't so keep in mind that everything works together for the good of your success. Exercise is very important and especially for one who is losing weight. You want to help tone your muscles and that can't be done just sitting around. Movement is important and so I teach low impact exercises to my seniors and handicap clients. They seem to enjoy the exercise more now since I have gotten them into the mood for doing them. Exercise can be fun if you take time to learn how to do it without causing pain or discomfort. I do recommend that you do at least 15 minutes of exercise a day. I now do about 30 a day in exercises and I got a dog recently and so walking she has become part of my exercise program. Many a day the dog walks me, but the point I am trying to get through to you is that exercise is very important so don't leave it out. Tone and stretch while you lose, and you won't have problems later.

Living with Fear

There is no cure for dealing with fear each person has their own way of conquering it. For some they face fear of the unknown head on without stopping or putting on the brakes. For others fear can be defeating and they withdraw often letting the fear over take them and their lives. For many like me fear is something you are afraid of but still challenge. I had all kinds of fears after I had my stroke. Fear that I wouldn't be able to lose the weight and that my heart would fail. I lived with that fear for months before I began to do anything about it. Just because you have fear in your life doesn't mean you will do anything about it. I had the fear of life being taken away from me but when it came to me eating and losing weight when I weigh over five hundred pounds, the fear just didn't seem that big.

Sure I heard the doctors tell me that I was endangering my life with each day I didn't do anything about my weight. But I had so much weight to lose that I just didn't know where to begin. More important it took years for me to gain the weight and I felt I would die before I was able to get it off. Especially since over the years I hadn't been able to lose and I had tried so many diets that I had lost count. Fear was eating me up inside I felt like I had no chance at success. I couldn't see how to get the weight off and I had hundreds of diets sitting in front of me to choose from. When you are that big you have to focus on something other than the weight itself. So I put my focus on food and making it taste good. I started conquering my fear of the unknown by reading and studying and asking a lot of questions. I wanted to know why people who had taken the trouble to lose the weight would gain it back. I didn't want to gain a pound back if I did lose it so I started asking questions.

I had a fear of being hungry so I would hold any menu up for ridicule. I knew eating that little would leave me hungry so I didn't start the diet. What changed was the way I began to see things. I first had to admit that I was scared of failing, but had more fear when it came to the unknown things I didn't know about weight loss. After reading numerous e-mails from people who had to stop the prepackage meals and found themselves gaining their weight back rapidly. I learned that prepackage is nice but that success comes from learning how to package your own meals.

I had a family who was eating with me so the meals had to satisfy all of us not just me. I found that the challenge came in learning to find meals for all of us to enjoy. One of my favorite meals to make for my grandsons are pizzas made from tortillas. I spread the tomato sauce and sprinkle the Italian seasoning on first. I then top the pizza with my treats or the family's specialty items. The last thing I add is a little cheese so that I don't go over my one ounce limit. I don't miss the extra cheese because I have replaced it with other things which take my focus off the cheese. This is something you might have to learn yourself but it can be taught and the benefits are rewards you will enjoy.

Fear can be what stops you from exercising you feel you will hurt yourself or not be able to do the exercise right. I had this fear I had been trapped on the floor for hours after falling so the thought of getting down on the floor to do any form of exercise was threatening. Even now I still harbor fears that I had embedded in me from the beginning. Even with the weight gone I still feel fear of maybe eating the wrong thing and the tube in my stomach becoming blocked. This fear is one you don't have to live with if you don't have the surgery. Some fears we can do without while others come with the territory. Nothing is full proof when it comes to dieting and that's what makes the whole thing obtainable. Once any fear is put under control you find you have the power to concur it. Fear can only destroy you when you don't take hold of it. I was afraid of control eating I thought it was a form of starving until I started practicing it. Once I began to recognize what a cup of something looked like and what I could eat and couldn't I soon lost the fear that control eating was bad. In fact I found that I became more controlled as I began to recognize that control eating was simply healthy eating.

I can truthfully say that I haven't been really hungry since I started controlling what I eat. In fact I often times cannot eat all that I is set in front of me in a serving. I try to stick to the basics and that usually fills me up. I usually can't eat all of the food at one sitting. I had a old weight watchers menu, one from my doctor and one from a prepared menu. I took time to look the items on the menus over and to find what was in common on all of them. I was surprise that most of the foods were identical only the way they served them was different. Where one had a hamburger Pattie, another called it hamburger steak, while another simply beef. The one thing in common was that they all said you needed 3ounces of meat. I found if I weigh up 4ounces and cook it then weighed it I usually had 3 ounces more or less. It wasn't enough for me to worry about. Most of the stress in dieting comes from worrying about something of little importance.

Does a fraction of a inch really matter when you have three hundred pounds to lose? The fear I had placed on the emphasis of the food soon lost importance when I began to learn more about what I was doing. I was learning to control myself through food and in doing so I was beginning to lose weight. Look at how many people find out they have diabetes and let the fear of the unknown override them. Diabetics have to learn healthy living in order for them to live. The fat which should not have been in the food in the first place has to be learned to be removed properly. They have to learn about herbs and spices and about controlled or proportion foods. So in fact they are blessed with learning how to live longer and healthier by changing their eating habits. Isn't that the same for anyone having to lose weight or change how they eat in order to live longer? Don't patients who have strokes or heart attack have to learn to eat healthy?

Healthy living is a way of life for so many of us today that the fear associated with it is beginning to disappear. Healthy living equals a longer life and that's something that we all want. Facing our fears is the beginning of the start of gaining success. Once you have the fear under control you will gain the strength you need to move forward. Success is as easy as learning to control that hidden fear. Any fear can be wiped out with time and education so start learning. Can a old dog learn new tricks? Yes, bark! Bark! I did!!!

My Bariatric View

Many people ask about my surgery and how it has affected my life. I cannot express this enough, that my weight loss was due to me learning how to correctly eat, cook, and proportion my food. I have learned a lot about weight loss mainly because of the fact this with this surgery come safety measures necessary for life. I was weighing in at 575 plus when I first went to Cori and asked for a consultation. I was told then that I would have to lose weight before they would consider doing surgery on me. I thought it was a bit much since I was going to them for help, so I left and decided against it. Mainly, because I didn't have the money to pay for the surgery. This was in 1999 when I began to develop severe muscle spasms and was having trouble walking. I had several other health problems but the fact I was losing my legs bothered me enough that I sought help.

I tried hard to lose the weight back in 1999 I went to several Healthy Living classes which were offered at the Community College. I took countless cooking classes to learn about how to properly cook the food. I took food handling courses so that I could learn how to properly care for the food. All of this was done in order for me to lose weight. None was lost. I was cooking healthy and loving it but I was still overeating so the weight was not coming off. I went on a liquid protein diet and it didn't work because I still didn't follow the program. I went to countless diet doctors and even went of the diet pills for a while. I lost a few pounds but once I stopped taking the pills I started gaining the weight back. I was becoming larger with each passing day and I just didn't understand why. One night I was watching the biggest loser on television and I listened to the doctor talk about food and exercise and their relationship to each other. I found myself so taken with what he was saying. He was hard on the people and they were listening and taking in what he said just like I was. The next day I decided to buy several books listing calories of the food we eat. I went to the local used bookstore and most of the books cost less than a dollar. Reading them began to put knowledge into my mind for I began to slowly understand why I wasn't losing weight but gaining.

I started measuring my food, but I was a complainer; I wanted to lose weight but I didn't want to do the work it took to get the weight off. I slowly began to come around and by then end of six months I had lost over seventy pounds. I have never gained those pounds back; I account that to the fact that I learned how to properly take the weight off by eating and exercising. By the time I went to Dr. T, I had already gotten my weight down to 338 pounds. I still had extremely high blood pressure and was having spasms so severe that I would become decapitated for hours, waiting on the spasms to end. Fear of losing my legs again sent me to the doctor, only this time the State of Michigan was willing to pay for the surgery. Now if at that time they would have told me that they wouldn't do all of the surgery needed for correction after losing the weight; I don't think I would have had the surgery. I feel that the surgery is a very good thing to have done if you are acutely obese or have severe health problems. I do not think that this surgery should be done just for beauty or vanity.

For one this is a very painful surgery which has threatening life problems if not followed correctly. I also found that there is no cut off point for this surgery, which the weight just keeps coming off. I am now a size 6 and I am worried that I will look sick or worse become sick from the weight loss. I eat 6 meals a day, just like in this program, but I increase the protein by adding protein powder in my cooking. I eat a great deal of extra protein because I am trying to tone up my thighs and arm; which took the most weight off and now I am left with sagging skin. I have about 8 inches on my arms and about 12 inches on my thighs. I am busy toning and trying to stretch my skin back to normal. This matter of sagging skin bothers me since all the while I was obese I was firm. I had nice firm breasts and now I have two deformed looking breasts. I have been training with weights and my breasts and my arms are beginning to look better but I have a long way to go.

I brought a machine which works on the thighs, but it hasn't changed too much other than making my behind sore. I have to remember the things I eat have to be chewed well. I don't want something to get lodged in my narrow stomach lining now. Only a person who has gone through the program and suddenly found themselves gaining their weight back will understand the importance of knowing proper food consuming. I have worked hard at my weight and I am working harder at firming. The one thing that the Bariatric program taught me is to walk. Only for someone obese walking isn't that easy. I learned to walk sitting down and within a matter of months, I had worked out a routine along with several others from my community; which began to slim me down. I couldn't walk standing up but I could go miles sitting down. I do sit up and leg up sitting down and I do many exercises in my bed. I wish that the doctors would have told me about all this sagging skin but never the less it's too late to quiver about it now.

So my opinion of bi-pass surgery is all good; if you are going to learn to eat properly; exercise and have enough money to have the correction surgery for the sagging skin. If though you are like me in a low income status and haven't the money to pay for the surgery; then your only alternative is to exercise and tone like me. I put on a pair of stocking and I look pretty good so thanks for the surgery; but no thanks to ever in life doing it again. I could have and would have gotten the weight off; because I was doing so I got off 237 pounds all by myself, by measuring and eating the proper amount of legal food. I found out all food is legal it's the portions which are dangerous if you over do them. If you choose to have the surgery then good luck and please learn portion control along with proper flavoring and cooking of your food.

I found that even with learning portion control and some heart healthy recipes that there was still so much more I had to learn. Bi-pass surgery leaves you always on edge about whether something might go wrong. Some of the proof now showing up in the medical reviews; lets us know that there is much more to learn about this surgery.

Consuming enough protein is important and find ways to do that is what makes it somewhat difficult for low income budgets. I found I was unable to purchase the protein powder like they suggest. I even tried to drink up the protein in breakfast drinks but couldn't afford that either. I found myself losing weight and becoming afraid that I wouldn't be able to consume enough protein. I stopped worrying one day when I thought about how I was losing the weight. I was eating healthy and feeling pretty good, in fact my skin and general health seem to be improving so I started counting protein that I was consuming and found that by adding protein at lunch and snacks I was just about where they wanted me to be.

I noticed that I was beginning to stable out and maintain a normal weight and that I also was beginning to fill out around my face. This made me happy but even more I realize that in eating healthy I was getting just that healthy and I haven't felt this good in years. The program of eating your way to a thinner you is design for anyone who wishes to follow the menus. The recipes have all been used by me over the four year period. You will notice that nearly every recipe is 300 calories or less a serving. This is for a reason so that you can consume enough calories that you will not become hungry. I hope that if you do decide to try this program you will find the method of eating fun and meaningful experience for not only yourself but the whole family. Healthy eating is for everyone and I welcome you to try and see don't you yourself enjoy the benefits it offers.

Breakfast Made Easy

I can't tell you how many breakfast's I created over the past four years but these are some which I found not only got me through but were easy to adjust to. Remember to check with your doctor to make sure you can follow the menus in this book.

Drinks That Satisfy

Popeye Special
1 cup of chopped spinach
(can use frozen but fresh gives the best flavor)
1 cup chopped strawberries
1 banana
½ cup shredded carrots
2 cups crushed ice

Blend all of the above ingredients until smooth. Thin out the smoothie by adding a little water. For added flavor you can add ¼ cup of plain yogurt. Diet sweetener to taste. I like flavoring with a little orange peel and 3 tablespoons of honey. Makes two serving; a great boost of energy for the person on the go.

The green color took some getting used to and to the dieter's which like putting a little protein in their morning try the following:

1 egg yolk
3 sardines

Add the following to the above ingredients but omit the yogurt. This drink is rich in vitamins needed to jump start any day. Be careful of the egg should be drank at one serving. Use less ice and water for a thicker drink.

Tropic Special
1 Banana
1 naval orange peeled and section
½ cup crushed pineapple (unsweetened)
5-6 strawberries
½ cup apple juice
2 cups crushed ice

Blend until smooth thinning as needed with water. Can sweeten with diet sweetener to taste. Make this drink a smoothie for a snack by adding ½ cup of plain yogurt. Makes two serving.

I like these two smoothies and recommend them for you to try mainly because they satisfy the taste buds. When you pick the fruit you like remember to try paring them with a vegetable and seeing whether you like the taste. Spinach combines well with most fruits but it is a taste that has to grow on most people. By adding the protein these drinks can be turned into a meal substitute.

Standard Breakfast Menu

This menu can follow most programs and it works well for all diet plans still check with your doctor

1 egg
2 ounces of meat

½ cup vegetable
½ cup of fruit
4ounces of skim milk or milk substitute
1 slice starch or ½ cup starch
Diet beverage drink

Sample Breakfasts
1 poached egg on a slice of dry toast
½ cup slice tomatoes
3 slices of turkey bacon
4 ounces of skim milk
4ounces of Orange juice
Coffee

1 egg beaten
2 ounces of chopped turkey ham
2 T. chopped green peppers
2 teaspoons chopped onions
Spray frying pan with non stick spray. Heat on medium
heat beat egg and add ham, pepper and onions and add
to pan. When edges form flip over to make omelet.
Serve with sliced pears and 3 slices of Melba toast.
Milk, coffee or tea finishes the meal.

Learning how to create meals that all the family will
enjoy is a matter of trial and error. This simple breakfast
roll up is liked by the entire family and is easy to make.
Double up on the recipes amounts the serving is for one
person

Mexican Egg rolls
1egg plus one egg yolk
2 ounces of ground sirloin
¼ teaspoon chili powder
¼ teaspoon cumin
¼ teaspoon garlic powder
¼ teaspoon onion powder
1 large tortilla

Mix the above ingredients together and fill the tortilla and roll up. Grill on a non stick skillet which has been sprayed with vegetable spray until golden brown. Serve with slice tomatoes and chopped mango. Try making a small
Smoothie without fruit for added flavor.

Yogurt smoothie

1 cup plain yogurt
1 teaspoon banana or vanilla flavor
½ cup of skim milk
1 cup of crushed ice

I started making this smoothie in-between meals when I felt a little hungry but had eaten my snack. I usually would get hungry right before lunch and I didn't want a large snack just something to hold me to my next meal. This simple drink did the job. I substitute different flavors but if I am really hungry I add a few tablespoons of fruit puree. This shake has saved me many a day and I hope it will save you too. It doesn't matter how you substitute as long as you start each day with breakfast. It is important to give the body some fuel once we wake up and that is true. The way we consume the fuel is up to us so if you like cereal eat cereal. If eggs please you eat eggs but don't overeat. If you stick to the basic breakfast menu you will find yourself eating a menu which satisfies and after a few weeks you will have adjust to controlled breakfast meals. Learning to substitute items is important you might find it helpful as I did to purchase some cookbooks which specialize in healthy eating. I found that the recipes for making breakfast were helpful in teaching me new things that I didn't know. I learned how to give breakfast a new twist and that's half the fun of learning when it comes to cooking. I now know how to make low calorie syrup and homemade sugar free jam. I can make omelets as well as muffins that are legal. Breakfast can be drunk or eaten but it has to be consumed at one's rising.

Make sure that you change over to turkey bacon and sausage as your breakfast meat. Bake or Broil all meats in the morning you do not need to consume fat first thing in the morning. For energy I would recommend you try eating fruits and vegetables they give an instant boost but remember like with sugar it crashes you out if you use all sugar and no substance. Protein is the fuel which keeps the body going it helps the muscles stay alert. Sugar fuels but it's the protein which keeps you really going. Now in between meals are the all important snacks and that will take you the most getting use to?

Snacks are designed to help get you through to the next meal. There are so many snacks out there and all of them claim to be healthy for you. I found that the only safe snack is one that I have created myself. I like calcium as a snack so I eat a lot of yogurt and cheese. There are so many cheeses to choose from and you can eat an ounce a day. I enjoy cheese and crackers with grapes. I also like matching cheese with flavored crackers. You can eat five of most crackers I tend to shy away from crackers that say you can eat more than ten. I like crunching on things so I like munching on carrots but I get a kick out of eating baked sweet potato fries. They are a terrific full of calcium and best of all they are sweet and I feel like I am cheating. I like using kosher salt but I try not to salt them at all I like using a vegetable spray on them and baking them on a high heat which causes the skin to get crisp and the potato to become even sweeter. I have even made carrot fries only they aren't as good but they're okay for a change of pace. When it comes to snacks it's a matter of what you like and what you need to sustain you. I found that if I stuck to the following snack menu that I usually got through to the next meal.

0

1 cup of fruit
1 cup of vegetables
1 starch
1 dairy

I stopped eating meat as a snack except for peanut butter. I eat 2 tablespoon of peanut butter with crackers or on a slice of bread. I even spread it on apples and celery. I found eating raw fruits and vegetables to be more filling than eating cooked when it came to snack time. I like the crunch but if you don't stick to the cooked vegetables. It is the amounts that help you maintain until the next meal.

I learned to make fruit and vegetable trays by using ½ serving of more than one vegetable or fruit. This variety helped breaks the routine and helped me to stay focus. I would substitute crackers and even learned to make homemade pita chips. I even know how to make my own baked potato chips. One potato sliced thin can add up to quite a lot of potatoes and when you flavor them with a little spice they really cut the hunger. Another snack which is great for helping you get through the day is homemade broth. I take chicken or chicken parts and cover them with water and bring them to a boil for fifteen minutes. I then cover the pot and let it steep and then strain it into container. I flavor my broth with Italian seasoning and a little cumin. I even put a pinch of cayenne pepper in it to add spice and a little black pepper for bite. I do not add salt. The broth can be drunk anytime and it has enough flavors that it cuts hunger especially when you add an ounce of cheese and five crackers. If you're hungry eat something or better yet try drinking the broth. A good tip to remember is the chicken used to make the broth makes a great oven fried chicken. The process of poaching the chicken first makes it moist when baked.

When it came to me accepting eating some many vegetables and fruits in one setting I just wasn't a happy trooper. I had to learn to accept that this way of eating could be done and have fun learning to do it. Because of my grandchildren I learned to enjoy gelatin. I use the sugar free brand and I found that just about all of them will adapt to fruit being added. I started a little cottage cheese with a little fruit in the flavored gelatin. One of my favorite ways of eating veggies is sautéing them until soften then letting them cool. I then add them to two packs of sugar free gelatin which has been mixed with 1 cup boiling water. I like using lime gelatin or lemon depending on the color of the vegetables. My grandson loves eating the veggies this way and so does my teenager. They say you forget that you're eating vegetables and I agree with them. Tired of eating veggies the same old way then try this and see if it becomes a family favorite for you too.

I had a problem with swelling feet so I began to eat more vegetables such as mushrooms or a cucumber which helps rid the body of water naturally. I found that eating a salad of cucumbers and mushrooms right before bed helped with swelling during the night. Following any program needs practice I would suggest that you practice eating snacks that you find enjoyable. Like anything if you don't like the snack or if it doesn't please you, you'll find yourself looking for something that does. Snacks are meant to help not to hurt or hinder you. Keep in mind you're eating your way to a healthier and thinner you.

Lunch is a very important meal of the day it is the second meal which holds us and gets us through to dinner. Though snacks are important they do not fuel the body with enough to get through the day. Lunch should be something special and should take some thought. When you don't plan your lunch well you can be sure your dinner won't satisfy you. It is the second meal which you will consume meat at and you also will increase your vegetables at this meal. Lunch is usually eaten at the high point of the day and it helps fuel the body for the rest of the day. I found that lunch works better if you don't weigh yourself down with too heavy a meat or anything to complicate. Lunch should be fun and satisfying not only to the taste but to the sight. To understand the importance of any weight loss program you have to understand how food works in the body. Because you have more time to burn off the calories you consume during lunch eating the heavier foods for lunch is a good idea. When I first started trying to lose weight I would eat my heavy meal at the end of the day. I would always feel stuff when it came time to go to bed. Mainly because by the end of the day; I didn't have enough time to work off what I had eaten. I would usually be tired from running around all day so I often times would fall to sleep. So I decided to change some things around in order to help myself get more control.

One of the things I changed was making my heavy meal in the afternoon or at lunch. I still suggest you follow the standard menu for dinner only the time changes. Casseroles are great to eat at lunch time they usually easier to consume. There are numerous casserole dishes which are low calorie and yet they are delicious. I personally like mixing all of my vegetables and meats together and forming something appealing and filling. I like cold casseroles as well as the hot ones but even better are the leftovers. When I had to carry a lunch to work I would cook the casserole the night before for dinner and take the leftovers to work with a salad and some fruit. Planning your meals ahead of time is important it allows you a chance to switch foods around. I had no idea how not planning was contributing to my failure. Lunch should be more than a sandwich or a burger it should be a culinary feast. A good trick is to set the table like you are at a restaurant and make sure when possible to include a guest.

You are more likely to stick to the program if you are sharing the meal with someone other than the television. I would invite friends over to try out a new recipe and they would be impressing with the table setting. So before you decide to sit down along try inviting a guest to share the meal with you. No one to invite don't let that stop you from treating yourself special. Put some flowers on the table and try using that special china that has been sitting on the shelf drawing dust. The extra effort you put forth will make you feel better and even make the food taste better.

The standard dinner menu is
4 ounces of meat
2 cups of vegetables
1 starch
2 cups of fruit
Salad
1 cup of calcium
½ cup chicken or vegetable broth

Remember a baked potato can be substituted with a cup of rice or noodles. I use milk or yogurt to bring a casserole together and vegetables can be mixed and matched to equal the total allotted amount. I tend to use beef or pork at lunch since they are heavier and it takes more for them to leave the body. I like using the lighter meats at the last meal of the day. If I fall to sleep I don't feel so bad if I had fish or turkey at the meal. If you notice I don't add fats to my meals I found that using chicken broth or a vegetable broth gave the food enough flavor that I didn't miss the fat. Fruit can be added to the salad or even put into sugar free Jello for a dessert.

A standard lunch menu would be
3 ounces of meat
1 cup of vegetables
1 cup of fruit
1 starch
1 dairy

I found the end of the day is a great time to enjoy a sandwich and some broth. A simple salad with meat can also be filling with fruit and yogurt as a dessert. The three main meals and three snacks should be spaced out three hours apart. The last meal should be eaten two hours before going to bed this allows the food time to digest. I once again I stress that I am no doctor that the information in this book was written in answer to the questions so many people have asked me over the last four years as I lost the weight. Many people asked me what diet did I follow and how was I am to stick to the program and reach my goal. I can only tell you the facts as I have lived them and thus the above menu is the program which not only helped me take off the weight but also helps me today to maintain my weight. When I first started the program I will admit I was hungry not because I wasn't getting enough food, but because I had to condition my mind that the food I was processing was more than enough to satisfy me. So that I wouldn't cheat or stop the program I would eat salads and drink the homemade broth in between meals with my snacks. I have made my homemade broth out of beef bones, chicken bones and parts, vegetables, ham bones to name just a few things. I always bring the mixture to a rapid boil for ten to fifteen minutes then cover and turn it off. I let it sit for thirty minutes before straining it and storing into containers. You can store the mixture for up to two days in a fridge but can store it for three months if kept in the freezer. I don't recommend storing it longer because the nutrients will have fallen off. This broth is made without salt but I do flavor it with the following before cooking: 2 teaspoon Italian seasoning, 2 tablespoon onion powder, 2 garlic powder or minced garlic, 1 teaspoon cumin, 1 teaspoon thyme, 1 teaspoon black pepper, and 1 teaspoon cayenne pepper. You can cut the cayenne pepper down to ¼ teaspoon if the above is too hot for your taste. I found that these herbs boost the flavor of the broth and gives it a wonderful smell as well as taste.

There is no full proof way to diet or takeoff weight everything in this book was tried and then tested before I accepted it as a daily routine in my life. I found it easier to stick to the program knowing I could add a little something extra helped me stay focus on reaching my goal and I hope that some of the tips will help you too stay focus and reach your goal. I can't promise anything because with myself I made no promises. I just kept to the program and by the second month the weight was falling off. I would concur my urges to eat sweets by eating fruit and by eating Jell-O which had fruit inside it. The fruit inside the Jell-O helped me to accept the amount of food I was in taking and stretching my meals to the next session. If you overeat you will not lose and if you under eat you will not lose. It takes a certain amount of food for the body to maintain and then to release the discarded fat.

When I didn't eat enough I wouldn't lose I simply held stationary. I found that eating was not enough that I had to exercise in order to burn more calories. Yes, you will lose if you don't work out but you will lose more if you increase the motion of your body in a workout. Do not over do this diet is to help you not to stop you from reaching your goal. I give you all of the tips I used to stay focus on the program and some that I picked up along the way. Learning how to make dishes I liked with the items on the standard menu was the challenge. I have enclosed several menus for you to follow or to help you plan your own. If you noticed I tried to get menus that gave big flavor but had few calories. I learned to cook my food with time and you will learn the same also. I find that maintaining on this program is easy simply because I have learned how to memorize the correct proportions. I cannot tell you how important measuring the correct amount is and learning how to recognize when you are overeating. I found that others will help once they know what you are doing and see the results of such. I had more people signing on to walk along side of me as I lost the weight. They too lost weight and learned how to eat healthy. Over the last two years I have tried this program out on numerous people and they have had results running from ten pound to twenty pounds of weight being loss the first month. You in general will only lose four to ten pounds a month, and for the most part you will only lose three to four pounds a month. I didn't give myself a set weight to lose that way I didn't leave myself set up for failure.

No doctor can tell you how much you will lose for certain or how long it will take. That depends on the person and how they stick to the program and especially how many calories they burn after consuming the food. If you simply wait on the food to react in your body you will lose a few pounds a month. For the big weight loss you have to give something in order to get to the goal. This program once again can be adjusted to meet everyone's needs in the family. I found that it was fun making a pizza which was healthy and not loaded with fat. I have made pizza with meat, vegetables and my favorite is a fruit pizza that I have brushed with a sugar free jam before serving. The jam gives it a shine which makes it more appealing. I used fresh fruit so the pizza wouldn't become soggy when cooking. My teenagers enjoyed eating the fresh basil and mozzarella pizza. They liked the fact they could personalize their pizza and still enjoy a healthy meal. In this day and age where our teens and children are gaining weight at an incredible rate it was nice to find something they enjoyed and was good for them too.

Don't push the menu at your family let them come into it on their own. You will find them joining in and eating along with you once they see how much fun you are having eating your way to a thinner you. Try making the fruit and vegetable trays with the fruits and veggies for the day and munch on them all day. Leave them in the fridge so they can stay cold and eatable. Nothing is full proof on a diet you can substitute and exchange foods all day as long as you stick to the program and don't add extra food. Learning to eat healthy is fun and I welcome you to try it and see don't you too get results that bring a smile to your face.

Remember a little stretches a long way in this program and learning to mix and match the food will enable you to stay focus and reach your goal weight.

Imagination is what helped me reach my goal weight and is what is keeping me maintained at that weight. I use my imagination in flavoring foods I try new herbs and spices regularly. Some I like and some I just don't I have learned to substitute Italian parsley or cilantro, mainly because I can't stand the taste of cilantro. If you have the same problem you might want to try the same and see how you favor it.

You have to experiment with the food until you get the right combinations and flavors that you and your family enjoy. I found that adding a little cayenne pepper or pepper seeds give the food a little heat but that heat also helps me when it comes to controlling my appetite. Just don't overdo or you'll pay for it later. If you happen to use too much pepper you can tone it down a little by adding a diet sweetener. Just don't overdo you don't want to ruin the dish completely. When adding pepper I add a pinch at a time until I reach my desired heat appeal. I like having gravy on my food so I learned to make a gravy substitute which for the most part satisfies the craving. I use 1cup of homemade chicken broth(can use low sodium canned broth) bring it to a boil, then add 1teaspoon of cornstarch mix 2 Tablespoons of hot water and2 tablespoon of light olive oil. Blend with whisk until thicken and serve immediately. This recipe has served over five people so don't consume all of it in one serving and never more than once a day. The reason I learned to make healthy gravy was for my family. They liked gravy on their mashed potatoes and I wanted them to enjoy one that wouldn't hurt them. Even in my gravy I add a pinch of pepper seeds for flavor. If you are craving something it is better to try to substitute it with something healthy but with the same see sight appeal.

If you are craving fried chicken a poached chicken will not end the craving. Oven fried chicken can be crunchy or soft it's all in how you apply the coating.

The recipes are in no special order the reason for this is to help you look through all of the recipes before choosing one. I had trouble with sticking to the menus until I started looking through all of them for something to eat. I found that my taste would change with each day and that I had fun looking through the recipes and finding something different. I don't like order when comes to food. I think you should be able to pick anything you like in reason and enjoy it.

Recipes, Recipes and More Recipes

The following recipes are in no order but they sure did help me get through the years of taking the weight off. I hope some of them will become favorites of yours and your family. Remember to stick to the standard format and enjoy as you learn to eat your way to a thinner you. Please remember to check that you can adjust my menus to your diet plan if you are diabetic. For bi-pass patients you can add the plain powdered protein to your ground meat to boost up the protein count.

Meatloaf

This meatloaf can be made with ground turkey, chicken, pork as well as beef. I use the correct amount of meat so that no matter what you substitute the flavor will be the same. This meatloaf is great in a sandwich and can be frozen for a meal another day.

4 egg whites
½ cup low fat milk
1 teaspoon garlic powder
½ cup Italian bread crumbs
½ cup chopped onion
½ cup chopped green pepper (can use red or yellow)
3 pounds of lean meat
1 tablespoon tomato paste
¼ teaspoon cumin
¼ teaspoon poultry seasoning
Pre heat the oven to 350

Combine the ingredients and mix well in a bowl. In a loaf pan which has been sprayed with a non stick spray put the formed loaf and cooks for 1 hour and fifteen minutes. Remove from oven and let cool for five minutes before serving. Cut into 4 ounce servings you should get anywhere from five to ten slice.

Per serving: 165 calories, 3 grams of fat, 1 gram of saturated fat, 14 grams protein

Though no salt is added there is salt in the breadcrumbs so watch your consuming. Serve with sliced carrots which have been cooked in ¼ cup of Splenda until tender. Mashed potatoes, which have been made with 1teaspoon of garlic powder and 1 teaspoon onion powder. I like using powdered milk which I control the water and white pepper to taste. Serve with broth gravy.

Crispy Baked Chicken
6 servings

2/3 cup of crushed rice cereal
¼ cup Parmesan cheese grated
1 tablespoon Italian bread crumbs
1teaspoon dried chives
1 teaspoon dried parsley
6 boneless chicken breasts
3 tablespoon of light olive oil
3 tablespoon of flour

Heat oven to 350
Combine dry ingredients in shallow dish. In another dish add oil and dip chicken in oil then in the dry ingredients and place on a baking dish which has been sprayed with a non stick spray
Leave room between meats so it can brown properly
Cook for 25 minutes or until no longer pink or bloody
245 calories per serving 35 protein grams

Cod in Tomatoes and Onions
4 6ounce cod fillets
8 tablespoons of light olive oil
½ red onions sliced thin
4 tomatoes chopped into medium cubes
¼ cup of sliced black olives
¼ teaspoon of dried thyme

1 teaspoon dried basil or 2 tablespoon fresh basil
1teaspoon garlic powder
Heat oven to 400

Rinse fish and pat dry dip in oil then sprinkle with dry seasoning lay in shallow baking pan top with remaining ingredients and bake until fork tender. About 15 minutes drizzle with remaining oil set sit five minutes before serving
245 calories 12 grams fat 31 protein grams

Lobster Lettuce Rolls
3 pounds of cooked lobster which has been shelled and flaked
¼ cup of reduced fat mayonnaise
1 celery diced and deveined
1 teaspoon lemon juice and 1 teaspoon lemon peel
4 large romaine lettuce leaves
¼ teaspoon garlic powder
¼ teaspoon onion powder
Pinch of cayenne pepper

Mix ingredients together in a bowl fill each lettuce leaf with a scoop full. Should line the entire leaf which is used as a bun. Can use a wheat bun for a sandwich.
200 calories 24 protein grams

Chicken Pizza
1 whole wheat thin pizza crust or 2 large pita breads
6 ounces of cooked chicken breasts cut into strips
½ cup of large mushrooms sliced thin
½ cup of sliced thin red onion

½ cup of green pepper sliced thin
½ cup of black sliced olives
1 cup of tomato sauce mix with
1 tablespoon tomato paste
1 cup low fat shredded mozzarella cheese
1 cup low fat cheddar cheese
Preheat oven to 375

Place crust of choice on a baking sheet which has been sprayed with a non stick spray. Top with sauce and remaining ingredients sprinkle the basil on top of the cheese bake for twenty minutes or until cheese is melted

Each slice is 210 calories Should get eight slices

Teens love this pizza it is good to make for school fairs and bake off's.

Chicken and sugar peas

1 tablespoon canola oil
2 tablespoon light olive oil
1 pound of chicken breast trimmed and sliced thin
1 teaspoon five spices
2 teaspoons minced garlic
1 pound of sugar peas clip ends
1 large carrot sliced thin
1 cup of whole mushrooms
1 tablespoon soy sauce
¼ cup of chopped green onions

Heat oil in large pot or wok to hot add the chicken garlic, dry ingredients and stir until tender. Stir constantly for about 4 minutes then add the sugar peas and remaining ingredients and cook until bean are fork tender about 4 more minutes top with green onions and serve over a scoop of rice

240 calories 30 grams of protein

Tropical Salsa
½ cup kiwifruit chopped
½ cup of mango chopped
½ cup papaya
½ cup of chopped pineapple
¼ cup green pepper
2 Tablespoons of chopped jalapeno pepper
1 tablespoon of lime or lemon juice
2 tablespoon of pineapple juice

Combine ingredients chill and serve about 60 Calories per serving

Peach salsa

1 teaspoon lemon peel
1 cup of chopped peaches (can use frozen)
½ teaspoon of chopped parsley

Combine well and chill before serving about 50 calories per serving

Lemon Pepper Catfish
1 ½ pounds of catfish fillets about a inch thick
1 teaspoon lemon peel
1 teaspoon black pepper
2 tablespoon light olive oil

Preheat the broiler spray pan with non stick spray

Rinse and pat dry the fish dip in oil then the peel and pepper mixture

Broil for 6 minutes or until fish flakes

150 calories 18 protein grams

Stuff Green Peppers

1 cup cooked brown rice

½ cup diced tomatoes

½ cup garbanzo beans drained

1 teaspoon Italian seasoning

¼ teaspoon black pepper

4 large bell peppers which have been cleaned out

½ pound of ground meat (cooked and drained)

1 tablespoon chopped garlic

¼ cup of crumbled mozzarella cheese

Preheat oven to 350

Combine all of the ingredients and fill the pepper shells with equal amounts and top with cheese bake until the cheese melts

Each pepper is 480 calories 43 grams of protein

Can served with a salad and fresh fruit

Herbed Chicken

1 cup chicken broth
½ teaspoon rosemary
1 teaspoon sage or poultry seasoning
1 teaspoon dried basil
1teaspoon dried parsley
Preheat oven350

Brown chicken place in shallow pan cover with broth and seasoning cook for 25-30 minutes until juice runs clear

285 calories 41 protein grams

Lamb Pita sandwiches

½ pound of boneless lamb culets
4 whole wheat pitas
¼ cup plain yogurt
2 tablespoon low fat mayonnaise
1 teaspoon dried dill
1 tablespoon minced garlic
1 teaspoon onion powder
1 small cucumber sliced thin
1 small tomato thinly sliced
1 small red onion thinly sliced

Preheat oven to 350

Heat pitas in fold and set to side

Put in a small bowl to chill yogurt, mayonnaise and dill

Heat lamb and remaining ingredients until done about 4-5 minutes

Stuff the pitas with equal amounts of the meat top with cucumber and tomatoes and topping

240 calories 12 grams of protein 4 servings

None of the menus are written in blood so if you want to change them around to suit your taste do so. I found these rubs to come in handy when flavoring meats like chicken and pork and it can be used to flavor turkey with some surprising results. I didn't add pepper seeds but you can add them to any recipe to spice it up a notch. Pepper is great for helping curb the appetite.

Indian Rub
1 tablespoon cumin
1tablespoon coriander
1tablespoon paprika
1 tablespoon ginger
1tablespoon turmeric
1 teaspoon cayenne pepper

Combine in a bowl and store in air tight container

Cajun Rub

2 tablespoon sweet paprika
2 tablespoon chili powder
1 teaspoon garlic powder
1 teaspoon onion powder
1 teaspoon oregano
1 teaspoon thyme
1 tablespoon cumin
1teaspoon black pepper
1 teaspoon cayenne pepper

Combine all ingredients store in air tight container

Herb rub
1 tablespoon rosemary
1tablespoon oregano
1 tablespoon thyme
1tablespoon marjoram
1 tablespoon basil
1 tablespoon fennel or anise seed
1tablespoon tarragon
1 tablespoon black pepper
1 tablespoon lavender leaves

Combine and store in an air tight container

When using rubs let the meat marinate for a half hour before cooking. Grilling this way gives the meat flavor as well as helps keeps in the moisture.

Banana Nut Bread
2 cups of flour
2/3 cup diet sweetener
2 ½ teaspoons baking powder
½ cup salted chopped nuts
2 beaten eggs
1 cup of mashed banana (about 2 bananas)
½ cup of vanilla soy milk
3 tablespoon light olive oil
1 teaspoon vanilla flavor

Preheat oven to350
Sift dry ingredient together in mixing bowl stir in the nuts

Combine the eggs, bananas, milk, oil and vanilla and add to flour ingredients pour into a sprayed loaf pan cook until the fork or toothpick comes out clean. One slice per serving about 120 calories Keep bread in the fridge for freshness

Great vegetables to grill indoors or out
Asparagus
Eggplant
Tomatoes
Mushrooms
Pineapple
Apples
Try serving grill veggies in sandwiches and in salads for added zest

Five great ways to get antioxidants into the system

Add berries to cereals
Snack on apples and pears
Toss a salad of spinach with olive oil
Add a few raisins to chicken or salad
Chop up some onions and add to salads and casseroles

Looking for a new pasta salad why not give this one a try

Tuna Pasta salad
8 ounce cooked pasta shells of choice
1 five ounce can of tuna drained
½ cup of low calorie mayo

1 cup of frozen peas thawed
½ cup diced carrots
½ teaspoon lemon pepper seasoning

Mix all ingredients well and chill serve on bed of lettuce

Simple Chicken Salad
1 4ounce can of chicken drained
1/3 cup of grapes sliced in half
¼ cup of chopped walnuts
3 tablespoon low calorie salad dressing

Combine all ingredients and chill serve on lettuce or with crackers

Need to create something in a hurry that the family will enjoy try

Chicken Rice Taco Toss

1 pack rice-a-roni
1 ½ tablespoons light margarine
1 16ounce jar of salsa
1 pound of boneless chicken breasts chopped
1 cup of frozen corn
4 cups of shredded lettuce
½ cup shredded cheddar cheese
2 cups of tortilla chips broken into pieces
1 medium tomato chopped

In a large skillet; sauté rice in margarine over medium heat until golden. Slowly stir in 2 cups of hot water, salsa, chicken and seasoning package. Bring to a boil then immediately reduce heat to low and simmer for ten minutes. Stir in the corn cover and simmer for ten more minutes or until chicken is done, Serve on top of lettuce top with chips and garnish with tomatoes

275 calories 23 proteins 6 servings

Need some simple tips for breakfast try some of these?

Quick cooking oats cooked with milk top with brown sugar and fresh berries. Can use dried fruit (great source of vitamin c and protein)

Make a breakfast parfait with fresh or frozen fruit which has been thawed. Layer with plain yogurt and top with crumbled graham crackers sprinkle with a little cinnamon

Make peanut butter sandwiches with bananas and serve with slice oranges sections or orange juice

Want to snack on something light for breakfast try an easy trail mix

1 cup of mini wheat cereal
½ cup of walnuts or almonds
¼ cup of raisins
¼ semi chocolate chips

Mix well and store in air tight container

In the mood for a Hero Sandwich try

6 tortillas

½ cup shredded lettuce

6 1ounce turkey slices

6 1ounce ham slices

6 1ounce Swiss cheese slices

2 small tomatoes sliced thin

11/2 cup bean sprouts

Arrange the ingredients on the tortilla and wrap in plastic wrap cut before serving

212 calories per serving

Got a sweet tooth try this apple pie

1 premade pie crust

3 apples peeled and cored and thinly sliced

1/3 cup of brown sugar diet sweetener

1 teaspoon cinnamon

1 tablespoon reduced fat margarine

¼ teaspoon nutmeg

1 tablespoon skim milk

1 teaspoon sugar substitute

Preheat oven to 350

Fill crust with apples and spices which has been combined with brown sugar dot with margarine and fold crust over. Brush with milk and sprinkle with sugar. Bake for 45-50 minutes

165 calories per serving

Having trouble knowing how much is a serving here some clues that might help out:

1 medium apple sliced thin ....2 servings
1 banana 8-9 inches long..............2 servings
1 cup of chopped broccoli............2 servings
¼ wedge of cantaloupe.................2 servings
6 baby carrots...........................1 serving
2 celery stalks...........................2 servings
16 grapes.................................1 serving
1 cup raw spinach.......................1 serving
½ cup zucchini...........................1 serving

It might be wise to buy a book which lists the proper serving amounts so that you won't overeat. It's easy to substitute once you know what to switch off with.

Need to switch off some snacks try:
Instead of fruited yogurt why not eat the following meal

½ small whole wheat pita
2 thin slices of turkey breast
1 slice thin tomato
Mustard to taste

Instead of 1 ounce of pretzels and ½ cup of grapes try:

½ whole wheat English muffin
1ounce of reduced fat mozzarella
3 thin slices of green pepper
3 thin slices of tomatoes

Instead of a breakfast bar try:
1 slice whole wheat toast
1 scrambled egg
2 slices of baked turkey bacon

Instead of trail mix try:
Whole wheat tortilla
1 thin slice of avocado
2 slices of chicken breast
1slice of tomato
Shredded lettuce
1 tablespoon salsa

Want a fruit salad that's easy to make try:
¼ cup mango
¼ cup watermelon
¼ cup cantaloupe
Serve on a bed of lettuce can top with
a little low calorie dressing

Try this Jamaican grill Chicken when you want something spicy

¼ c jar chutney
1 teaspoon pepper sauce
4 boneless chicken breasts
2 tablespoon Jamaican jerk seasoning

Preheat grill to medium high heat
Combine pepper sauce and chutney and set aside
Rub chicken with seasoning and grill for seven minutes or until done brush with the chutney
200calories per serving

You can pull together some mouth watering meals with these pantry items:

Brochette mix can be stirred into pasta for a light snack, or toss with lettuce and toasted bread cubes for a quick panatela salad

Garlic paste can be added to ground meat for added flair

Sun-dried tomato pesto can be added to cream cheese for a quick dip or to marinate a piece of poultry

Use hoisin sauce for a quick dip for grilled veggies or for a glaze for chicken or pork

Try using a chutney stirred into some yogurt for a change of pace

Season rice vinegar and canola oil and a little soy sauce makes a great dressing for salad
orcestershire sauce wakes up the flavor of grilled mushrooms or sprinkle on roasted potatoes for added taste

Need some speedy side dishes

Bulgur has a nutty flavor and cooks up in 20 minutes ouscous is ready in 5 minutes and can be made to taste even better by adding lemon zest, chopped basil or dried herbs

Try microwaving some rice in 2 minutes and adding frozen peas to boost the vitamins

Quinoa is ready in 12-15 minutes and can be served with soy sauce, sesame oil or lemon juice

Try almonds in food for added crunch they add protein, fiber, and vitamin E to a meal. They are also good for those watching their cholesterol level

During these times when stretching the buck is at the top of the list try some of these three dish recipes:

Caribbean wings

1 pound chicken wings
1 cup of chopped mango
3 tablespoon mango puree
¼ cup hot sauce

Combine all ingredients and put on a baking sheet bake for 25-30 minutes or until done makes 4 servings

Spicy tortilla chips

8 soft corn tortillas
¼ cup dark chili powder
2 tablespoon ground cumin

Cut the tortilla into wedges. Spray tortilla chips with non stick spray. Bake in 350 oven for 3-5 minutes sprinkle with seasonings.

Basic Granola

1 cup whole wheat flour
3 cups rolled oats
1 cup brown sugar substitute
16 tablespoons of light olive oil
½ cup water

Preheat oven 300

Combine dry ingredients. Whisk together the oil and water and pour over dry ingredients. Spread out on baking sheet and bake for 25-30 minutes or until crisp. Store in air tight container. Makes 8 serving

Easy Chicken Cacciatore

2 green peppers sliced thin
1 chicken cut into quarters
1 jar mushroom tomato sauce

Preheat oven 350

Combine ingredients together and bake in shallow pan for 45 minutes or until done

Chicken stuffed with Feta and Spinach

10 ounces of fresh spinach
2 ½ pounds of chicken breasts washed and dried
8 ounces of feta cheese
2 tablespoon margarine

Preheat oven 400

Flatten chicken breasts with rolling pin or pan. Put a little feta and a handful of spinach on chicken and roll and pin together with toothpicks. Place in baking dish and spray with non stick spray and sprinkle with pepper bake until done about 25 minutes melt margarine and drizzle on chicken before serving

Roasted Turkey Breast with orange and soy dressing

1 small turkey breast
1 cup of soy sauce
2 cups of unsweetened orange juice

Preheat oven 325
Put turkey in roasting pan with sauce and juice and bake for 2 to 21/2 hours basting with juice.

Glazed Short Ribs

3-4 pounds of short ribs trimmed of all fat
2 cups of Teriyaki sauce
1 cup of Hoisin sauce

Put all of the ingredients with 3 Tablespoons of garlic powder, 2 tablespoons of onion powder into a bag and marinate for 3-4 hours to overnight. Preheat oven to 350
Put ribs into a casserole dish that has a tight fitting lid. Can use a slow cooker for this dish. Cook for 2 to 21/2 hours until the meat is tender and baste the meat with the liquid you marinated it in until the meat has absorbed the sauce and left a light glaze. You should remove the lid after 2hours and continue the glazing for up to an hour and served with a salad

Cabbage soup

1 medium cabbage chopped or thinly sliced

½ can of diced tomatoes
½ sliced thin white onion
4 cups of low sodium chicken broth
¼ teaspoon dried parsley
¼ teaspoon garlic powder

Bring all ingredients to a boil, then turn down and simmer for fifteen minutes. This is a very low calorie soup and can be used as a snack or in between meals to help trim the appetite

Chicken Noodle Soup

½ chicken cut into parts and boiled and cooled and shredded
1 large carrot sliced thin
1 celery stalk sliced thin
1 medium onion sliced thin
2 tablespoon minced garlic
2 teaspoons dried parsley
½ cup whole wheat thin noodles or shells
4 cups of low sodium chicken broth

Bring all ingredients to a boil and then simmer for 30 minutes or until the carrots are tender. The soup is considered a meal because of the meat inside. It can be substituted for ½ meats and ½ starches in the exchange.

Spiced Up Chili

1 ½ pound of ground meat, browned and drained on paper towel
1 medium chopped onion
1 medium chopped green pepper

2 tablespoon of minced garlic
2 tablespoon of cumin powder
2 tablespoon of chili powder
1 teaspoon cayenne pepper
1teaspoon black pepper
1 can of kidney bean rinsed
1 large can of diced tomatoes
1 tablespoon dried basil
3 cups of chicken broth

Bring all of the ingredients to a boil and turn down and let simmer for an hour and a half. This chili takes time you want to cook it until it is reduced and thicken. You can a 1 teaspoon of diet sweetener if it is a little to bitter. It taste better the second day and is always considered ½ of your meat exchange to one bowl. I use turkey, chicken or pork as the meat when I want to lower the calories. Add 1 tablespoon of poultry seasoning and 1 teaspoon Italian seasoning for flavor.

All three of these soups taste good and are better the second day. Serve them with a salad and some floating bread cubes for a variety or change. Remember you can only have one bowl of the Chili a day. I again say I am not a dietitian but if you check with your doctor you will see that the foods are legal. I recommend that you make sure you can have them before starting to incorporate them into your diet.

Basic Meatballs

1 pound of ground meat
1 egg
1 cup of season breadcrumbs
2 tablespoon of olive oil

Combine all the ingredients in a mixing bowl. Add 1 tablespoon of garlic powder, 1 tablespoon of onion powder, 1 teaspoon black pepper and combine well. Make 2 inch balls of meat and place into a shallow baking pan and bake at 350 for 45 minutes. Can serve these balls with gravy or tomato sauce and served on 1 cup of rice. Three balls of meat is one serving if they are 2 inch balls.

Tasty Burgers

1 onion chopped
1 pound of ground meat
2 tablespoon of Worcestershire sauce
1 teaspoon garlic powder
1 teaspoon onion powder
1 teaspoon poultry seasoning

Combine well all the ingredients and form into patties. Place on a cooking sheet or shallow pan which has been lined with foil. Cook in a preheated oven 350 for 30-35 minutes or until the meat is done. Serve with a salad and lettuce and tomatoes.

Cajun Burgers

1 pound of ground meat
1 tablespoon of Cajun spice
1 tablespoon on garlic powder
1 teaspoon onion flakes
1 teaspoon of black pepper

Combine the ingredients well and bake in a preheated oven 350 for thirty to forty minutes or until the meat is done. Serve with baked sweet potatoes fries and a salad

Drunken Burgers

1 pound of ground meat
1 tablespoon of grill seasoning
½ cup of light beer

Combine all the ingredients well and cook on the grill or can pan fry until the burgers are done. Makes four regular burgers goes good with a salad and baked fries

Meat Pie
1 pound of ground meat
2 cups of roasted tomatoes
½ cup of corn (drained)
½ cup of salsa
1 box of corn muffin mix
½ cup of cheddar cheese

Preheat the oven to 350

Combine the meat and all ingredients except corn muffin mix

And pour into a baking dish. Make the muffin mix as directed and pour on top of the meat and top with the cheese and bake for 20 minutes or until the cornbread is done. Toothpick should come out clean.

Baked Corned Beef
1 corn beef
2 tablespoon of dill or pickle spice
1 cup of Dijon mustard

Preheat oven 325

Simmer the meat in a covered pot for 2 hours then put the meat into a roasting pan and bake for 11/2 hours or until the meat is done. Sauce should be poured over the meat when done and served with Cole slaw

Easy Corn Beef Hash
1 pound of cooked corn beef
which has been cut into cubes
1 bag of frozen hash browns (diced and cubed only)
2 onions diced
1 green pepper diced

Combine all ingredients well and put into a baking dish and bake in a preheated oven for 20-30 minutes or until potatoes are tender. Serves 4-6 people

Roasted Veal
1 veal round roast (4pounds)
¼ cup chopped rosemary (3 tablespoon of dried herb)

10 pears cut in half

Preheat oven to 350

Rub the roast with olive oil and season with black pepper before putting in a roasting pan. Cut the pears and put them around the roast. Sprinkle the roast and the pears with the spices and bake for 40 minutes or until done. Serve 8 people

Simple sauce for meat
1 cup of wine (can substitute apple juice or chicken stock)
2 Tablespoon margarine

Heat the wine until hot and whisk into the wine 1tablespoon of margarine at a time until it melts. Serve the sauce over the meat enough for 6 people

Tasty sauce for Meat
½ cup of water
2 tablespoon of honey
3 tablespoon of cider vinegar
1 tablespoon of sugar substitute
1 tablespoon of Dijon mustard
2 tablespoons of chopped tarragon
1 teaspoon of minced garlic

Combine all the ingredients and whisk with 1 tablespoon of cornstarch. Bring to a simmer over medium heat and serve over meat. Chill the leftovers for another day.

Black Stew
In a slow cooker
1 pork shoulder
2 cups of black beans which have been drained
2 cups of green salsa

Rub the pork shoulder with olive oil and season with black pepper, garlic powder and onion powder. Place the meat into the slow cooker and add the remaining ingredients. Cook for 2-3 hours until the meat is tender. May need to add 1 cup of water during the cooking keep an eye on the cooker do not let it dry out.

Baked Pork Chops in Mustard Sauce
2 pounds of pork cutlets
½ cup of Dijon Mustard
1 tablespoon of grill seasoning
1 cup of season breadcrumbs

Preheat oven to 350

Season the meat with seasoning dip in mustard and into the breadcrumbs. Place the meat on a shallow baking pan which has been sprayed with a non stick spray. Leave a little room around the chops so they can brown evenly. Bake for 40 minutes or until the meat is done.

Green Peppers and Pork chops

3 medium green peppers sliced thin
6 pork chops
½ cup of apple cider vinegar
1 large onion sliced thin

1tablespoon minced garlic
1 teaspoon black pepper

Preheat oven to 350

Place all ingredients into roasting pan make sure the meat is covered well. Cook until done roughly 40 minutes serve over brown rice with a salad

Fruity sausage and onions

1 medium onion chopped fine
2 apples sliced thin
1 pound of sausage links
1 teaspoon all spice

Preheat oven350

Put all the ingredients together in a baking pan and bake for 25 minutes until apples are tender but not overcooked

Roasted Lamb
11/2 cup of flour
2 tablespoon of thyme
2 tablespoon of rosemary
1 leg of Lamb
1tablespoon black pepper

Combine all the ingredients into a bowl and rub over the lamb place in a roasting pan. Cook the meat until done at least 30 minutes. Meat will have a light crust serves 6-8

Lamb Burgers

1 pound ground lamb
1teaspoon rosemary
1 teaspoon thyme
1teaspoon onion powder
1teaspoon garlic powder

Combine all ingredients well and form patties Bake in a preheated over 350 for twenty minutes Makes 4 patties

Lamb Curry

1 pound of onion chopped
2 pounds of chopped lamb meat
1 8ounce can of curry sauce

In a slow cooker
    Place all ingredients and bake on low heat until the meat is done about 11/2 to 2 hours. Serve with basmati rice and a salad. Serves 4

Lemon Salmon

1 whole salmon gutted and scaled
3 Tablespoon of dill seasoning
7 lemons sliced thin

Combine all ingredients and let marinate for 3-4 hours. Place on grill and cook for 15-20 minutes Lemons should be tender and the Salmon should flake. Wrap salmon in foil with lemons to keep warm until you serve with rice and salad. Cut salmon into 4-6 serving.

Basil Poached Fish

½ cup of chopped fresh basil
1 cup of white wine
4-6 fish fillets

Lay the meat in a preheated fry pan cover with wine and basil and bring to a simmer with a lid until fish is tender and flakes about 10-15 minutes. Drizzle the sauce over the meat before serving

Steamed Shrimp with Beer

2 pounds of shrimp with shells
1 bottle of light beer
1 tablespoon of grilling seasoning
1 small onion sliced thin

Combine all ingredients in a fry pan with lid Simmer until shrimp are pink 10-12 minutes do not overcook drizzle with olive oil before serving makes 4 serving

Italian shrimp

2 pounds of shrimp peeled and deveined
2 cups of pasta sauce
1 cup of Parmesan cheese
½ cup of season breadcrumbs

Top the shrimp in the pasta sauce and then breadcrumbs and place in a casserole dish. Broil in the broiler for 10-12 minutes then top with the cheese and broil for 5minutes or until the cheese melts 4 serving

Easy Peach Cobbler

1 pound of peaches
1 cup cinnamon sugar (1 cup sugar substitute plus 3 teaspoon cinnamon)
1 box of biscuit mix

Preheat oven to 350
Cover the peaches which have been sliced and quartered in saucepan for 15 minutes. Let cool. Combine all ingredients together and pour into a baking dish. Make the biscuit mix and spoon over the peaches. Bake for 20 minutes until the biscuits are done and golden brown

Peanut Butter Cookies

1 egg
1 cup of peanut butter (better if you use nutty peanut butter)
1 cup of sugar substitute

Preheat oven 350
Beat the eggs and then add the remaining ingredients together and drop on to a baking sheet which has been sprayed with a non stick cooking spray. Bake for 6-8 minutes let cool for 5 minutes before removing from tray to a cooling rack Makes 24 cookies

Orange Tea

2 cups of orange juice (unsweetened)
2 cups of tea(strong brew is best let cool)
¼ cup of diet sweetener

Combine and serve over ice with lemon slices. Can add ½ cup of rum or vodka for a spiked tea

Apricot Chicken

½ cup of lemon juice
¼ cup of Dijon mustard
2 teaspoon minced garlic
½ teaspoon white pepper
½ cup of olive oil
6 medium chicken breasts
3 tablespoon cornstarch
1 can unsalted chicken broth
1cup apricot preserves
2 teaspoon margarine
1 cup of sliced almonds

Marinate the chicken in the lemon juice, mustard, garlic, pepper, and ½ cup of olive oil. Let marinate for 3 hours. Remove the chicken and place in a large heated skillet and cook for 8-10 minutes or until the juices run clear. Combine the broth and cornstarch with a whisk until smooth. Stir in the butter and a little of the marinade until it is thicken. Spoon over the chicken sprinkle with the almonds which have been lighted toasted and serve over rice.

Balsamic Chicken Salad

6 chicken breasts cut into 3 inch strips
1 teaspoon minced garlic
4 tablespoon olive oil
¼ cup balsamic vinegar
11/2 cup of cherry tomatoes cut in half
1 tablespoon of chopped basil
1 tablespoon of dried basil
¼ teaspoon pepper
6 cups of spring greens

In a large skillet sauté chicken, and garlic until the chicken runs clear when pierced. Add vinegar, tomatoes, basil and pepper; bring to a boil about five minutes. Put the chicken over the spring greens and serve immediately. 6 servings 226 calories 24 proteins

Sausage Soup

4 cups of water
1 potato diced small
6 turkey sausages (browned and diced)
2 cans of kidney beans
1 can of diced tomatoes
1 medium chopped onion
1 medium green pepper chopped
2 bay leaves
½ teaspoon garlic powder
½ teaspoon black pepper
½ teaspoon thyme

Combine all ingredients in a pot with lid and bring to a boil. Turn down and simmer for 10-15 minutes and take out the bay leaf. Serves 10-12 people 1 cup of soup equals 160 calories 10 protein grams

Cheesy Ham Pasta

8 ounces of uncooked pasta
1 pound of process cheese
½ cup nonfat milk
3 tablespoon ketchup
2 cups of ham cooked and diced into cubes
1 package of frozen peas
Preheat oven 350

Cook the pasta. In a medium saucepan add cheese and milk and heat until smooth. Add in ketchup and combine with ham and pasta and peas. Bake for 30 minutes serves 4

Sweet and Sour Chicken Wings

1 medium green pepper chopped
1 onion thinly sliced
1 tablespoon canola oil
1 can of unsweetened pineapple chunks
3 tablespoon white vinegar
2 tablespoon soy sauce
2 tablespoon ketchup
1/3 brown sugar substitute
2 tablespoon cornstarch
12 ounces of cooked chicken breasts cubed

In a large skillet or wok stir fry the peppers, onions until tender. Drain the pineapple keeping the juice for later. Add 1cup of water to the juice, vinegar, soy sauce, and ketchup add to above ingredients and bring to a boil. Combine brown sugar and cornstarch in a separate bowl slowly add to the mix slowly until thicken. Add the pineapple reduce the heat and simmer uncovered for 5 minute. Serve over rice. Makes 4 serving

Mashed Potatoes with sauerkraut

2 2/3 cups of water
2/3 cups of milk
¼ cup margarine cubed
2 2/3 cups of mash potato flakes
1/3 onion chopped
½ cup sauerkraut drained
4 turkey bacon strips crumbled

In a large saucepan combine the water, milk, margarine to a boil. Stir in potato flakes and let stand for 5 minutes. Brown onions until tender stir in the sauerkraut and potatoes and mix well. Serve with the crumbled bacon on top of potatoes. Makes 5 servings

Spanish rice

1 small onion chopped
1 tablespoon margarine
2 cups of uncooked instant rice
1 can of tomatoes diced
1 can of green chilies drained

1 cup of water
¾ cup of beef broth
½ teaspoon chili powder
¼ teaspoon sugar substitute
¼ teaspoon cumin

In a large saucepan sauté onion in margarine until tender. Add rice and cook and stir for 2 minutes. Stir in tomatoes, water, broth, chili powder, sugar, and cumin. Bring to a boil reduce heat and cover and simmer for 5 minutes. Remove from the heat and let stand for 5 minutes Makes 4 serving

1 cup of rice is 258 calories

Herb Steak fries
4 cups of frozen steak fries
1 tablespoon olive oil
11/2 dried basil
11/2 dried parsley flakes
¼ teaspoon garlic powder
¼ teaspoon paprika
¼ teaspoon black pepper
¼ cup of Romano cheese

In a large bowl combine the everything but the cheese. Combine well and arrange on a baking sheet which has been sprayed with a non stick spray. Bake in a preheated oven450 and bake for 20 minutes or until browned and sprinkle with cheese. 4 servings

Bean and Cheese Quesadillas

4 flour tortillas
2/3 cup refried beans
11/2 cup of cheddar cheese shredded
¼ cup of chopped green chilies
1/3 cup of sliced green onions
1/3 cup of sliced black olives
1 cup salsa

On two of the tortillas spread refried beans, sprinkle with ½ cup of cheese, top with chilies, onions, olives then top with the rest of the cheese and add the remaining tortillas. Cook over medium heat or grill pan for 4 minutes until browned and cheese is melted. Cut into wedges and serve with a spoon of salsa. 2 serving

Easy Broccoli Slaw

1 package of broccoli coleslaw mix
3 ounces of dried cranberries or cherries
6 green onions chopped
¼ cup of coleslaw dressing mix

In a large bowl combine the coleslaw mix, berries and onions. Toss and refrigerate makes 8 ½ cup servings

Guest Beans and Mushrooms
3 turkey bacon strips diced
3 cups of fresh mushrooms sliced
¾ cup chopped onions
¾ cup sweet red peppers(can use green)

4 cups of frozen green peas thawed
¾ teaspoon pepper
¼ teaspoon garlic powder

In a large skillet cook bacon over medium heat and set aside. Stir in the mushrooms, onions, peppers and sauté for 8 minutes or until the vegetables are tender. Stir in the peas and remaining ingredients reduce the heat and simmer for 4-5 minutes until heated through. Crumble the bacon on top before serving.

Makes 6 servings

Veggie Muffins

1 cup of flour
1 cup of cornmeal
1 tablespoon dried parsley
1 tablespoon dried basil
11/2 teaspoons baking powder
1 teaspoon oregano
2 eggs
1 cup of winter squash thawed
¾ cup of plain yogurt
¼ cup olive oil
1 cup frozen corn
2 green onions chopped

In a large bowl combine the first seven ingredients. In another bowl combine eggs, squash, and oil. Stir in the corn and onions. Coat the muffin tins with non stick spray the fill each tin with an ice cream scoop of mix. Bake for 15-20 minutes until toothpick comes out clean. Cool for

5 minutes before removing to cooking rack serve warm. Makes 12 muffins each muffin is 160 calories roughly.

Spicy Broccoli Pasta with Ham

8 ounces uncooked pasta (can use any pasta)
21/2 cups frozen broccoli spears
1 medium onion sliced thin
1 teaspoon minced garlic
2 cups of ham which is cubed
1 can of sliced black olives drained
¼ cup olive oil
½ teaspoon Italian seasoning
½ teaspoon crushed red pepper flakes
½ cup of Parmesan cheese

In a large saucepan cook the pasta add the broccoli, onions and garlic during the last 7minutes. Cook unit the pasta and the broccoli is tender. Drain. In a large serving bowl add the pasta and all the remaining ingredients. Sprinkle with the Parmesan cheese right before serving. 4-5 servings

Remember that when you cook dishes which have the meat and starch together that you must measure out properly you're serving. Do not overeat the dish simply because you have used more than one item. This diet works well if you stick to the proper measuring tools and don't cut them short. The above recipe can be served with a salad and fruit.

Easy Sloppy Joes

1 pound ground meat
½ cup chopped onion
½ cup condensed tomato soup
½ cup unsweetened ketchup
3 tablespoon unsweetened grape jelly
1 tablespoon brown sugar substitute
1 tablespoon cider vinegar
1 tablespoon mustard
½ teaspoon celery seeds
5 whole wheat rolls or buns split

In a large skillet cook ground meat with onions until the meat is browned. Drain. Stir in the remaining ingredients and bring to a boil before reducing the heat. Simmer uncovered for 15 minutes and scoop with ice scooper on to the buns. Makes 5 servings

Speedy Chili

11/2 pounds of ground meat
2 small onions, chopped
½ cup chopped green pepper
1 teaspoon minced garlic
2 cans of kidney beans drained (can omit)
2 cans of stewed tomatoes
1 bottle of light beer (can omit)
1 small can of tomato paste
¼ cup chili powder
¾ teaspoon dried oregano
½ teaspoon hot sauce

¼ teaspoon sugar substitute
¼ teaspoon black pepper

In a large pot cook the beef, onions, peppers, garlic until brown and drain. Add all the remaining ingredients to the meat and bring to a boil. Reduce and simmer for 20 minutes. Makes 12-15 1 cup servings

Any day Pork Chops

1 tablespoon brown sugar substitute
¼ teaspoon garlic powder
4-1inch thick pork chops
1 tablespoon olive oil
1 can of Mexican corn drained
11/3 reduced sodium chicken broth
1 pack of cornbread stuffing mix
2 tablespoon unsalted butter

Combine the brown sugar, garlic powder, and rub over the pork chops. In a large skillet brown the chops in the oil on both sides and remove and place on paper towel. In the same skillet combine the corn, broth, stuffing mix and butter. Top the pork chops and cover and cook for 15 minutes or until the meat tender. Makes 4 servings.

Bean Salad

1 can butter means drained and rinsed
1 pint of cherry tomatoes- halved
1 small red onion chopped
½ cup of diced yellow squash

½ cup diced zucchini
¼ cup fresh parsley chopped
Dressing
3 tablespoon olive oil
2 tablespoon lemon juice
1 teaspoon cumin

In a large bowl combine the beans, tomatoes, onion, squash, zucchini and parsley. Combine the dressing ingredients and add to the bean mix and gently toss. Cover and chill. Makes 6 serving 1 cup is 120 calories

White Bean Soup
2 small zucchini quartered and sliced
1 cup chopped onion
1 cup chopped celery
1 cup chopped carrots
2 tablespoon canola oil
3 cans unsalted chicken broth
1 large can of northern beans which have been drained and rinsed
1 large can of white kidney beans which have been drained
1 large can of diced tomatoes
½ teaspoon dried thyme
½ teaspoon dried oregano
¼ teaspoon black pepper

In a slow cooker sauté the zucchini, onion, celery and carrots in the oil until tender. Add the remaining ingredients and bring to a boil then simmer for 20 minutes covered or until all the veggies are tender.

Meatball Soup

3 cups of frozen green beans
2 cups of baby carrots
2 cups of low sodium chicken broth
1 teaspoon dried oregano
1 teaspoon dried basil
1 teaspoon minced garlic
2 cans of stewed tomatoes
16 turkey meatballs
2 cups frozen corn

In a large saucepan or soup pot combine all of the ingredients and bring to a boil. Reduce the heat and simmer for 15 minutes. Meatballs for this soup can be made the day ahead try this simple recipe.

Meatballs
1 pound of ground meat (can use any ground meat)
½ cup of season breadcrumbs
½ teaspoon parsley
½ teaspoon poultry seasoning

Mix well all the ingredients and form 1 inch balls and bake in the oven for 20 minutes. Can freeze for use later for up to three months. Meatballs can be spiced up by adding:

½ teaspoon hot sauce
½ teaspoon pepper flakes
1 teaspoon Italian seasoning

Make the meatballs small this is a great appetizer. I like simmering the meatballs in ¾ cup orange juice it adds zest and the flavor is exceptional.

Mexican Soup

1 tablespoon canola oil
1 small onion chopped
1 jalapeno pepper diced
2 tablespoon minced garlic
2 teaspoons cumin
5 cups of low sodium chicken broth
11/2 pound boneless chicken breasts cut into cubes
2 cups salsa
2 tablespoon black pepper

Heat large saucepan over medium heat. Add the onion and pepper and cook until tender. Stir in the garlic and cumin and then add the broth stirring well after adding. Bring to a boil then reduce to a simmer. Add the salsa and all of the remaining ingredients. Simmer for 10 minutes and serve hot.

Zucchini Soup

2 teaspoon olive oil
1 small onion chopped
1 teaspoon minced garlic
2 medium zucchini sliced thin
1 tablespoon ground ginger
1 teaspoon curry powder
3 cups of vegetable broth

½ cup of plain yogurt

Sautee onions and garlic until soften. Add zucchini, ginger, curry powder, and continue cooking. Add the broth and bring to a simmer until the vegetables are tender. Stir in yogurt before serving.

This soup has a lot of flavor and can be frozen for up to two months. You can add a extra curry powder to taste and if you want to spice it up add 1 teaspoon of pepper seeds.

Greens and Bean Soup

1 bunch of Swiss chard with the stems removed can use
Mustard greens in place of Swiss chard
2 teaspoons olive oil a little extra for drizzling on soup
before serving
2 stalks of celery chopped
1 small onion chopped
1 tablespoon minced garlic
3 cups of low sodium vegetable broth
1 can on diced tomatoes
1 large can of navy or white beans
½ teaspoon oregano
½ teaspoon black pepper

Add all the ingredients in a large soup pan and bring to boil. Simmer for 10 minutes and serve immediately

This soup can be thicken by adding ½ cup croutons and drizzling a little olive oil on top before serving.

Baked Sweet Potato Fries

2 medium sweet potatoes slice and dried
1 tablespoon of olive oil
¼ teaspoon pepper
½ teaspoon paprika
Preheat oven to 400

Toss the potatoes in the oil and sprinkle the seasoning on them and layer on a cooking sheet. Bake for about 15 minutes then turn over and continue to bake for another 10 minutes. Serve the fries hot. Can sprinkle with kosher salt or for a sweeter potato sprinkle with diet sweetener once you take them out of oven.

Easy Cole Slaw

1 cup low calorie mayonnaise
3 tablespoon Dijon mustard
3 tablespoon apple cider vinegar
1 teaspoon sugar substitute
1 small cabbage shredded thin
1small red cabbage shredded thin
1 teaspoon black pepper
1 teaspoon garlic powder
1 teaspoon onion powder

Whisk together mayonnaise, mustard, vinegar, sugar substitute. Add to the cabbage and toss well to combine. Add pepper and chill until ready to serve.

Pear Tart
1 tablespoon lemon juice
1 tablespoon sugar substitute
¼ teaspoon cinnamon
½ teaspoon almond extract
3 medium pears cut and sliced thin
6 sheets of whole wheat phyla dough thawed

Mix ingredients together and layer the fruit between the dough spraying each sheet with non stick cooking spray. Fold the edges together and bake until pears are tender and crust is golden. Best when served warm or right out of the oven.

No diet will work if you are not willing to cut back and learn to cook the food without all the fat. Learning to eat the proper amount will lead to you not only eating healthy but will enable you to lose weight. Our goal is to cook good food with a lot of flavor and still lose as we eat and enjoy it.

Almond Pilaf

¾ cup chopped onion
½ cup of slivered almonds
1 tablespoon unsalted butter
2 cups of low sodium chicken broth
2 cups of instant rice
½ cup frozen peas
¼ teaspoon black pepper

In a large skillet sauté the onions and almonds until tender in the butter. Add the broth and bring to a boil. Stir in the rice, peas and pepper. Cover and remove from heat and let stand for 10 minutes.

Polish Sausage Stew

4 cups of peeled potatoes cut into cubes
1 pound of polish sausage cut into 1 inch pieces
½ cup chopped onion
½ cup chopped green pepper
½ cup chopped red pepper
11/2 teaspoon Cajun seasoning
3 tablespoon olive oil
½ cup of baby carrots
1 bay leaf (remove after cooking)

In a large skillet heat all of the ingredients until fork tender. Can add ½ cup of chicken broth if you like gravy or to help tenderizer the vegetables. Makes 6 serving

Beef and Spaghetti

1 small zucchini cut into 1inch slices
1 teaspoon minced garlic
1 tablespoon olive oil
11/2 cups thin sliced cooked sirloin beef
¾ cup of cherry tomatoes cut in half
¼ cup low calorie Italian dressing
Cooked Spaghetti for two

In a large skillet sauté zucchini and the garlic in olive oil until tender. Add the beef, tomatoes, and the salad dressing and heat until the beef thoroughly warmed. Served over the spaghetti and sprinkle with a little parmesan cheese before serving.

Cauliflower and Tomatoes

1 pack of frozen cauliflower thawed
6 slices of turkey bacon crumbled
1 cup season breadcrumbs
3 medium tomatoes
2 stalks of green onion chopped
1 teaspoon dried dill
¼ teaspoon black pepper
¾ shredded cheddar cheese

Cook cauliflower until tender. In a large skillet cook bacon and crumble. Toss the bacon and breadcrumbs in bacon dripping can add 1 teaspoon olive oil to moisten. Toss the cauliflower with the remaining ingredients and top with the bacon mix. Bake in a preheated oven 400 degrees for 10 minutes uncovered. Sprinkle with cheese and cook another 8 minutes or until the cheese is melted. Makes 6 serving

Stuff Tomatoes with Chicken

4 medium tomatoes
1 rotisserie chicken skinned and cubed
½ cup shredded carrots
¼ cup chopped green onions

1/3 cup low calorie mayonnaise
1/3 cup low calorie ranch dressing
¼ cup chopped walnuts (can use almonds)

Scoop out the tomatoes making sure not to puncture the skin. Add the remaining ingredients together and spoon into the tomatoes. Sprinkle with nuts and serve

Legal Club Sandwiches

½ cup low calorie mayonnaise
4 slices of thin slice wheat bread toasted
1 cup of shredded lettuce
8 thin slices of tomatoes
½ teaspoon black pepper
12 strips of turkey bacon cooked and drain on paper towel
½ pound of sliced thin turkey breast
½ pound of thin sliced honey baked ham
4 slices of Swiss cheese
1 avocado sliced thin

Spread the mayonnaise over the bread. Layer the lettuce, tomatoes, avocado, bacon, turkey, and ham. Add the cheese and top with the wheat bread toast. Cut in half and enjoy this is a complete meal so remember not to add anything other than fruit and something to drink.

Crunchy Strawberry Salad

1 package of ramen noodles broken into small pieces
1 cup of chopped walnuts

¼ cup olive oil
¼ cup diet sweetener
2 tablespoon red wine vinegar
½ teaspoon soy sauce
6-8 cups of romaine lettuce torn into pieces
½ cup green onions chopped
2 cups of fresh strawberries sliced

Heat noodles and walnuts in a skillet until tender. Drain. In a tight fitting jar add the oil, sugar, vinegar, soy sauce, and shake well. Add to the remaining ingredients and toss lightly. Serve immediately.

Shrimp and Linguine Salad

¼ cup olive oil
2 tablespoon white wine vinegar
2 tablespoon chopped fresh parsley
1 teaspoon cayenne pepper
½ teaspoon dried oregano
1 pound cooked and deveined shrimp
1 package of linguine
½ pound of frozen asparagus cut into pieces

Dressing
2/3 cup olive oil
2/3 cup Parmesan cheese
½ cup lemon juice
1 tablespoon lemon peel
½ cup chopped fresh basil

In a plastic bag add shrimp and the following ingredients vinegar, parsley, cayenne pepper, oregano seal and mix well and set aside. Cook linguine in the last 3 minutes add asparagus and cook 2 more minutes. Add all ingredients except basil and toss and chill. Sprinkle with basil right before serving.

Watermelon Salad

10 cups of seedless watermelon
2 pints of cherry tomatoes
1 medium red onion chopped
½ cup fresh chopped parsley
½ cup fresh chopped basil
¼ cup lime juice (can use lemon juice)
In a large bowl combine all ingredients and chill until serving.

Lemon Herb Chicken

1 cup of lemon juice
2/3 Italian salad dressing
2 teaspoons dried basil
1 teaspoon dried thyme
½ teaspoon black pepper
1 chicken clean and quartered

Combine all ingredients in a bag and let marinate for 4hours. Grill chicken until juices run clear basting with marinade while cooking.

This chicken is great in a salad the second day and makes a great sandwich.

Apple Flavored Country Ribs

¾ cup unsweetened apple juice
½ cup of light beer
½ cup canola oil
¼ cup brown sugar substitute
1 tablespoon Worcestershire sauce
1 tablespoon minced garlic
1 teaspoon dried thyme
1 teaspoon black pepper
½ teaspoon cayenne pepper
3 pounds of boneless country ribs

Combine all ingredients in a bag and let marinate overnight. Grill the ribs over medium heat for 30 to 45 minutes until tender and the juices run clear. Baste with the marinade serve immediately.

Hungry but can't figure what to eat? Well why not try something different like this Black bean chili. It's one that the whole family will enjoy and it's a welcome change to the regular chili. Stick to one bowl per serving but if you are still hungry after the first bowl you can have a half bowl more. (Roughly ½ cup). Make it fun night and fill some side bowls with the family favorites for topping the chili. Sour cream, chopped red onions, grated cheese, tomatoes, is just a few toppings. My family likes the homemade tortilla strips as a topping. Serve with large tortilla chips and make the chili a dip.

Black Bean Chili
Makes 8 serving

3 (15 ounce) cans of drained black beans
1 large onion chopped
2 tablespoon olive oil
4 teaspoon chili powder
1 teaspoon cumin
½ teaspoon pepper
1 pack of meatless burger crumbles
1 14 ounce can of chicken broth (can use homemade)
2 cans of chopped tomatoes
1 jalapeno chopped

Combine all of the ingredients in a slow cooker or Dutch oven and let simmer until all of the veggies are tender. This chili is high in protein and is good for bi-pass patients.

Creamed Turnip Greens

2 tablespoon olive oil
2 tablespoons minced garlic
1 (16 ounce) bag of turnip greens (taste better with greens from the garden
½ cup of homemade chicken broth
½ teaspoon of cayenne pepper
2 tablespoon of flour
1 cup of skim milk
5 ounce of cream cheese chopped into pieces

In a large skillet heat olive oil and sauté onions, garlic until tender. Add turnips and chicken broth and cook until the greens are tender. (5-8minutes) Sprinkle the greens with the flour and sauté a few minutes more. Stir in milk and cook until thicken 3 minutes, then add the cheese and stir until melted and serve immediately. These greens are a welcome change and small children will find them to be a delight on their plates.

Pecan Crusted Pork Cutlets

1 pound of pork tenderloins
¾ cup bread crumbs
½ cup finely chopped pecans
2 teaspoon sage
2 teaspoon onion power
2 teaspoon garlic powder
4 tablespoon olive oil
2 large eggs beaten

Stir together the breadcrumbs and pecans with seasonings. Dip the chop in the beaten egg and then into the breadcrumb mixture, Cook in the hot olive oil over medium heat until the juices run clear. Drain on paper towel before serving

Holiday Roast

1 -5 pound eye of round roast
2 tablespoon minced garlic
1 tablespoon of dried rosemary
2 teaspoon black pepper
2 teaspoon of oregano
1 large can of tomato sauce

½ cup of red wine
1 large chopped onion
3 tablespoon of flour
1 cup of beef broth

Place roast on a large sheet of foil. Cut slits into the roast then combine all of the ingredients forming a paste. Pour over the roast and cover and close tightly. Put in a slow cooker and let simmer overnight cook roast until tender and juices run clear. Let stand five minutes before serving.

Zesty Lemon Rice

1 teaspoon minced garlic
2 cups of chicken broth
2 tablespoon olive oil
1 cup basmati rice
1 tablespoon of lemon zest

Combine all ingredients together (except lemon zest) in sauce pan bring to a boil then reduce and simmer for twenty minutes. Add the lemon zest and serve.

Chinese Green Beans

2 pounds of frozen green beans
6 slices of turkey bacon chopped
½ cup sugar substitute
½ cup red wine vinegar

Add green beans to a saucepan simmer until tender. Add the bacon and the sugar and vinegar and bring to a boil in separate sauce pan. Stir occasionally for 5 minutes then add the beans and toss together serve over brown rice.

Holiday Salad

Cut cold cornbread into 1 inch cubes and place on a light sprayed aluminum pan. Broil for 6 minutes turning once for browning. Let cool then add to medium bowl of spring greens, add 3 ounces of chopped turkey strips or chunks. Add a few dried cranberries and or whole cranberries from the can to decorate. Serve with an oil and vinegar or Italian light dressing.

Once again I mention that I am not a doctor and nor am I a dietitian; I am simply a woman which lived most of her life overeating and not knowing anything about healthy eating. I don't want the recipes in any special order, nor do I want the information in any order. This book was meant to make you the reader, look and search through the pages looking for yourself something that only you can enjoy or understand. I lost by searching and learning and you will too. I hope that I have included something which will help you and yours reach your weight goals. I decided I would break here and speak more on the importance of exercise in relationship to dieting.

Exercise Tips

First and foremost let me say that exercise into a regular schedule is crucial for weight loss. The best exercise routine depends on the person and what they are willing to do. A good point to remember is that when it comes to weight loss you must burn more calories than you consume. Exercise will make your heart stronger, cause weight loss and lower your blood pressure. Here are some tips that helped me out and I hope they will help you out as well.

1. Ten minute of mowing the lawn, or gardening, or simple house cleaning is great exercise and is beneficial for your health.

2. Walking ten minutes whether you walk outside or do they sit in the chair exercises for walking, for at least 5-6 days a week will help in improving your general health. It requires no equipment, can be done at any time and any place and is one of the less-taxing exercise you can do and you will see results.

3. You have to learn to do movement so that you are burning calories throughout the day. Something as simple as taking a walk during your lunch period at work, or as just standing while talking on the phone at home will burn calories. Keep in mind the more calories you burn the more you will lose.

4. Weight training is important in rebuilding the muscles in your body. You can do the resistance training and achieved great results. You will not see the scale move if you do weight training but you will see your muscles become leaner and firmer. Having leaner body mass causes a person to burn more calories quicker.

5. Whatever it is in order for an exercise program to work you must be successful at doing it daily. You have to commit to it and remember that with pain comes gain; you will see the weight loss on the scale and the improvement in your health.

Now with all exercise comes the treat afterwards for all the effort you put into achieving it. Here is a great recipe I found for bread pudding I have made some changes so that you won't find the bread pudding showing up on your back side.

Fruit and Pudding Delight

1 cup of mixed raisins
½ cup of dried cherries
1 cup of dry wine (your choice)
1 large granny smith apple (cored, diced and chopped)
2 large pears (chopped, and diced)
1 tablespoon of unsalted butter
1 cup of brown sugar substitute (packed tight)
3 cups of fresh bread crumbs (use multi-grain bread)
4 cups of soy milk (vanilla flavor is best)
1 teaspoon of vanilla extract
¼ teaspoon of ground cardamom
3 large eggs
2 teaspoon of lemon zest
¼ teaspoon of fine sea salt (can use a salt substitute)

Combine raisins, cherries and wine in a shallow container and soak for at least four hours or overnight. Melt the butter in a saucepan, add the diced fruit and sugar and bring to a boil. Reduce the heat and simmer uncovered for about five to ten minutes. Allow to cool for about an hour or at least to get room temperature. In a large bowl, stir together eggs, lemon zest and salt. Whisk in the milk and vanilla and cardamom, add 21/2 cups of bread crumbs and let soak for an hour. Place oven rack on the middle and preheat the oven to 400. Spray with a butter non stick spray your pan (9x3 inch) sprinkle the remaining bread crumbs into the pan. Combine the bread mixture and the soaking raisins and fruit. Pour into the prepared pan and place on a baking sheet. (This helps if it overflows in the oven) Bake in a preheated oven for an hour; or until the pudding is evenly golden brown. You can serve this dish with sauce or yogurt with honey.

This recipe is 292 calories per serving and it is worth the trouble. It is also diabetic and bariatric friendly.

I love giving tips that I have learned that help keep myself fit and will do the same for you. Here are five things which will keep you on track:

1. Burn more calories as you unload the dishes from the dishwasher, why not set the table up for the next meal.

2. Try shopping or browsing the stores for bargains. This keeps you moving and is great fun for the whole family.

3. Write out your grocery list on an envelope and put all of the coupons you plan on using inside of the envelope.

4. Remember to keep all of your doctor appointments. Try to get the first appointment of the day; or right after lunch it saves on the time sitting there in the doctor's office all day.

5. Remember to treat yourself to something good so that you won't feel cheated. Remember that healthy eating is something the whole family can profit from.

I found that carbs can be confusing so here is a simple list you might get some help from:

Instead of white rice why don't you give brown rice a try

Instead of your bowl of corn flakes why not try bran flakes instead

Change from white bread to multigrain bread

From orange juice to a orange (a squirt in the eye is always fun)

From a baked potato to trying sweet potato

From plain pasta to a whole wheat grain pasta

Instead of applesauce try eating the apple

Another great tip is instead of three large meals why not break the meals down as I suggest and have six small meals. This is a great way of keeping on track and it fulfills the requirements of most diets. If you stick with healthy choices this approach can cut out or at least down the hunger pangs and help keep blood sugar levels steady.

I found that I was missing having my Banana pudding so here is a great substitute that worked for me:

Banana Cups

½ bananas thinly sliced
1 pack of (100 calorie Lorna doones)
2 packs of the sugar free or reduced calorie vanilla or banana pudding)
2 tablespoon of Light cool whip (can be left out)

Mix and prepared all ingredients then get some great cups or champagne glasses and layer each with banana slices and the cookies and then the pudding. Follow the layering until all of the glasses are full then top them with cool whip right before serving. Make sure you keep this dish cool until serving. The calories are only about 150 per serving and the taste is great. It is a beautiful arrangement that will help keep you on track and fill that sweet tooth.

Desserts can still be divine when you have diabetes or are a bariatric patient. You only have to modify them so that you will be taking the calories out and putting the flavor in.

Here are ten ways you can sneak in activity into your life:

1. Try going inside the gas station to pay for your gas.
2.
   Walk your family animal around the block.

3. Walk around the house while talking on the phone instead of sitting down.

4. Walk the stairs instead of taking the elevator.

5. Bring the groceries into the house one bag at a time.

6. March in place while watching television or do some sit down exercises while watching television.

7. Play with your grandchildren outside or find a outdoors sport you can enjoy.

8. Go inside the bank instead of going through the drive thru.

9. Ask a neighbor to go walking with you.

10. Dance while preparing dinner instead of watching television do so sit down exercises.

Before you laugh remember that these might seem like small things but everything adds up when you are burning calories.

I love good lasagna and here's one that the whole family will love and it diabetic and bariatric friendly:

Cheesy Meat Lasagna

¾ pound of lean ground meat
3 cloves of garlic minced
11/2 teaspoon of dried oregano
1 jar of spaghetti sauce
9 lasagna noodles cooked and drained
1 16 ounce low fat cottage cheese
2 cups of shredded reduced fat mozzarella
1 large tomato chopped

Preheat oven to 375

Brown the meat with the garlic and oregano in a medium saucepan. Stir in the spaghetti sauce and let simmer for 5 minutes. Remove from heat and stir in the tomatoes. Spread ½ cup of the sauce mixture in a 13x9 inch baking dish. Layer 3 noodles, 1 cup of cottage cheese, ½ cup of the mozzarella cheese, and 1 cup of the remaining sauce. Continue until you reach the top of the pan and cover with foil. Bake 30 minutes or until it is heated through. Uncover top with the remaining cup of mozzarella cheese. Bake uncovered for another 5 minutes or until the cheese is melted. Let stand 5 minutes before serving.

A good tip to remember is that if it says its low calorie it doesn't mean it isn't fattening. Watch your intake of food which says low or reduced calorie so that you won't find the scale moving upward.

Free Foods

Any food that is 20 calories or less and 5 grams of carbs is considered free food.

Diet beverages are free but they have tons of sodium in them so beware.

Veggies are considered free but watch out for over doing them you don't want to have a problem with gas later.

Remember that bouillon or broth is considered a free food but they too are high in sodium.

Fruits and Veggies

1 medium apple, orange or peach
1 small banana or ½ large bananas
1 cup of berries
Canned fruit in its own juice but keep it at ½ cup or less
½ cup of corn
12-15 grapes
1 cup of melon chunked
½ cup of peas
1 small potato baked
½ cup of sweet potatoes mashed

Grains

1 slice of bread
¾ cup of dry cereal
4-6 crackers (use the unsalted crackers)
½ cup of oatmeal
2 small pancakes
½ cup of pasta
3 cups of popcorn (unbuttered)
¾ cup of pretzels
1/3 cup of rice

Occasional Treats

2 inch square brownie
2 inch square of cake
1 small bag of chips (unsalted)
2 small cookies
1 frozen juice bar

½ cup of ice cream (try frozen yogurt
or a sugar free ice cream)
½ cup of pudding
¼ cup of sherbet or sorbet
1 small doughnut (plain)

These are only some of the items I tried and found acceptable in a trade off for something special to treat myself after a good day of dieting.

If you eat a lot of beans and you're looking for another way to serve them why not try this Lima bean casserole.

Lima bean Casserole

3 garlic cloves thinly sliced
1 tablespoon of olive oil
1 small onion chopped
¾ cup chopped carrots
8 ounces of ham cut into chunks
1 16 ounce can of butter beans
½ 16 ounce packages of frozen butter beans
21/2 cups of chicken broth (low sodium)
1 teaspoon of dried rosemary
Cornbread crust batter

Preheat the oven to 400

Sauté garlic in hot oil over medium heat for about a minute. Add onions carrots and cook until tender. Add ham and cook for another 4 minutes. Stir in the beans, peas, and the next two ingredients and bring to a boil and cook for 5 minutes. Remove from the heat and pour the cornbread batter over the mixture. Bake for 30 minutes or until golden brown and bubbly.

Cornbread batter topping
1 cup of cornmeal mix
½ cup of buttermilk
¼ cup of sour cream
1 large egg
½ teaspoon of dried rosemary

Combine all ingredients and pour over the bean mixture and bake immediately.

Remember that nonstick pans and skillets will help cut down on the oil and calories.

After a hearty meal why not try walking or doing some sit down exercises about ½ hour after eating. Here are some tips that might help out when it comes to posture.

Posture: walk with the head erect and the stomach pulled in.

Arm swing: bend your arms at a 90 degree angle and pump them gently as you walk.

Stride: step forward with your heel and roll off your toes. Stride should be natural so don't force it.

Speed: Be sure you can carry on a normal conversation and breath. It's no use in trying to win a marathon right off. Remember slowly and easy will always will the race when it comes to good health.

I know many people haven't tried Kale but this Kale and Potato Soup is one the whole family will be enjoying.

This soup doesn't take long to prepare and it's packed with flavor.

Kale and Potato Soup

1 bunch of Kale (roughly 1 pound)
2 pounds of boiling potatoes
1 teaspoon salt substitute
1 tablespoon of chopped onion
2 quarts of boiling water

Remove the stems from the Kale, wash the leaves and cut them into small shredded pieces. Peel the potatoes and chop them up very fine.

Bring the water to a boil and add the potatoes and onion and return to a boil and cook for 2 minutes covered. Add the Kale and cook for 2 more minutes. Adjust the seasoning and enjoy the soup.

In the mood for a great Potato Salad

¾ cup of mayonnaise (use a light or diet mayonnaise)
1 teaspoon of mustard
1 teaspoon of original Mrs. Dash
4 cups of boiled potatoes
¼ cup of chopped onions
½ cup of chopped celery
1/3 cup of green pepper chopped
2 hard boiled eggs chopped
1 tablespoon of dried parsley
¼ cup of pickle relish (can use ¼ cup of chopped pickles)

½ teaspoon minced garlic
1 teaspoon salt substitute

Wash and peel the potatoes and boil until tender. Rinse and cool potatoes and cut into cubes. Set aside. Place the onions, celery, green pepper, eggs, and parsley in a bowl. Add the salt substitute, Mrs. Dash, mayonnaise and relish. Mix well and add the potatoes and lightly toss until well mixed then chill for 1 hour before serving.

This salad is only about 185 calories to the ½ cup serving.

Remember it is easy to become overwhelmed. So try to pick out only one thing you do well and stick to it for the day. Change your routine each day so that you won't become bored and lazy.

Sample Menu

Breakfast
2 eggs scrambled lightly
2 teaspoon low fat butter (no salt)
2 sliced of baked bacon
1 small chopped red pepper
½ cup of chopped mushrooms
1 tablespoon of low fat cheese

Morning Snack
1 ounce of roast turkey
3 carrot sticks
1 cup of low fat yogurt
½ cup of fruit of your choice

Lunch
6 ounces of water packed tuna drained
1 tablespoon of low fat mayo
1 cup of shredded lettuce (try spring greens)
1 medium apple chopped
4 cherry tomatoes halved
1 cup of sliced cucumber

Afternoon Snack
1 cup of sugar free Jello
1 cup of low fat yogurt
½ cup of fruit of your choice

Dinner
6 ounces of boneless chicken breast
1 tablespoon of pesto sauce
1 cup of frozen green beans
1 ounce of low fat cheese
1 medium tomato

This menu is low in calories and shows how you can enjoy a lot of food and not feel cheated in the process.

Exercise is important here are some you can do laying in your bed:

1. Lie on your back with your legs in the air at a 90 degree angle
2. Rest your hands lightly behind your ears so your elbows point straight out to the sides.
3. Curl up so that your head, neck, and shoulder blades are off the bed. Use your abs not your arms to pull yourself up. Lower yourself back down and

repeat slowly for at least five to ten counts. You can increase as you get the hang of the exercise.

4. Lie on your back and bend your knees and slowly reach over the knee to the count of five. Do ten to fifteen but don't overdo you will feel the burn.

5. Lie on your back and lift both legs upward to the ceiling and slowly back down to the bed. Do fifteen and then wait for the count of ten and do fifteen more.

Still want something different for breakfast try:
½ small whole grain bagel
1 tablespoon of light cream cheese
Coffee, tea with ½ cup of low fat milk

1 cup of plain low fat yogurt
1 cup of berries

Remember to switch to a multi-grain or whole grain when it comes to starch. Fiber is important so don't leave it out just remember to monitor what you are consuming.

Snacks are important and can be fun try:
Hard cooked eggs
Raw jicama, bell peppers, or carrots sticks
Small apples or pears
Decaf cappuccino with fat free milk
Sugar free pudding
Fat free microwave popcorn
5-6 whole wheat crackers

1 cup of celery with 2 teaspoon of almond butter
Reduced calorie granola bar
¼ cup of chocolate covered soy nuts

Remember that dark chocolate has been proven to lower the blood pressure but don't overdo it.

6 ounces of fat free instant hot cocoa made with water
1 cup of raw broccoli
½ large grapefruit
1 small banana
1 cup of light yogurt
1 cup of ready to eat fortified cereal
11 dry roasted almonds
1 cup of red bell pepper
1 tablespoon of peanut butter

As with any snack you should stick to the amount you know is legal. It will only put calories on your backside if you don't!

Get creative when it comes to dinner try:

Beef Papikash- substitute 1 tablespoon of smoked paprika for the cumin and the coriander and parsley for the cilantro.

Sour cream spuds- Substitute ½ cup of fat free sour cream for the buttermilk.

Mediterranean Beef- Reduce the cumin to 1 teaspoon substitute 1 teaspoon of oregano for the coriander and 2 cups of green beans for the corn.

Substitute ½ cup of chicken broth for the buttermilk and 1 ½ teaspoon Olive oil is a wonder drug and it can make a potato come to life try:

An extra virgin olive oil.

For a fluffier and tastier potato reheat the spuds in the pan stirring constantly until dry. Add the liquid ingredients then mash with a potato masher and don't worry about the lumps they add to the dish. Try leaving the skins on for more nutrients.

Need to perk up your vegetables try adding lemon or orange zest on cooked green veggies. Added after cooking perks up the flavor and doesn't affect the color.

When you dine out at a restaurant don't order a cocktail out of habit. Try drinking a diet coke or soda first. When the meal arrives if you still want a drink order one then.

Stash a low calorie treat in your purse so if you get hungry you won't cheat. Dum-dum lollipops are great for this idea. I found you can nibble on two and not hurt your diet.

If sweets are on your mind try this recipe:

Butterscotch Bars

½ cup sugar substitute
½ cup brown sugar substitute
¼ cup of unsalted butter soften
2 large egg whites
1 teaspoon vanilla flavor
1 ¼ cup all purpose flour
½ teaspoon baking powder

¼ teaspoon salt substitute
½ cup of butterscotch morsels
Cooking spray

Preheat oven to 350

Beat sugars and butter with a mixer at medium speed until well blended. Add egg whites and vanilla and beat well. Lightly spoon flour into the dry measuring cups and level with a knife. Combine the flour to the sugar mixture beat at a low speed until blended. Stir in the morsels

Spread evenly into a 8 inch square pan which has been sprayed with cooking spray. Bake for 30 minutes or until a toothpick comes out clean. Cool bars in pan on a wire rack. Cut into 16 bars and enjoy 1 or 2 bars as a treat. Each bar is about 142 calories. Don't eat more than 2 in one day!

People getting on your nerves and you want to get rid of some stress. Try this knockout move:

Extend the arm out one at a time keeping your fist tight. Arms should be at shoulder and ten to fifteen of these jabs will relieve you of some stress that could otherwise cause you to cheat. I often think of someone who I would really like to punch out and my workout becomes more fun and I feel much better. Can't hit the real person but in your mind you can really knock them out!

Being overweight put you at risk for fatty liver disease, which interferes with the liver's ability to break down cholesterol.

Chest pain isn't the only heart attack sign. Women may experience indigestion, nausea, difficulty sleeping, shoulder or jaw pain, or shortness of breath.

You don't have to be overweight to have a heart problem so have the doctor check you out. Even better buy a blood pressure monitor and take your pressure every day. It is a good way to stay on top of a dangerous problem.

Menopause is fun at All!!! Here are some natural ways for getting a little relief:

Black Cohosh

St. John's Wort

Ginseng

Flaxseed

These four things helped me out and if you experiment with them they might give you a little relief.

Soy is good for you

Don't like soy beans why don't you try tofu, milk, cheese, yogurt or edamame. It is a good source of keeping the bones in tune but it is also a great way to keep those flashes under control.

Here's a real knee shocker!

If you've always wanted to take up jogging to spur your weight loss efforts but worried that it might cause knee pain, here is some good news that you may not have heard of. A new study shows that jogging may prevent osteoarthritis of the knee. A condition in which the loss of cartilage causes stiffness and pain. Jogging helps build muscle and boosts cartilage volume, both of which prevent the cartilage loss responsible for OA. Need another reason to hit the track? The calorie burning effect. One of the best ways to avoid OA is to get to-or stay at a healthy weight. Just remember to check with your doctor to make sure that this sport would be advisable for you.

Hot Pizza Surprise

3 cups whole wheat egg noodles
10 ounces of fresh mushrooms sliced
1 large bell pepper cut into strips
1 onion chopped
½ pound of lean ground meat
1 ½ cup reduced fat spaghetti sauce
1 large can (10 ounces) of cream of chicken soup
¾ cup of shredded cheddar cheese
1 3ounce package of turkey pepperoni
2 tablespoon reduced fat grated Parmesan cheese

Preheat oven to 350

Spray a 2 quart baking dish with a nonstick spray. Cook noodles rinsed and drain. Spray a nonstick large skillet with a nonstick spray. Cook the mushrooms, bell pepper, onions over medium heat for about 5 minutes. Add the meat and cook until browned. Add the spaghetti sauce, soup and the cheese and noodles. Spoon into the baking dish; and bake until hot for about 50 minutes then top with remaining cheese and the remaining ingredients. Bake about 5-7 minutes longer.

This dish is great for parties and for potlucks but you can even score a touchdown with it during the football games.

Cocoa Powder to the rescue

If you want a chocolate punch without blowing your diet try unsweetened cocoa powder. 1 Tablespoon of cocoa contains ¾ grams of fat while ½ ounce of unsweetened chocolate roughly the same amount contains 7 ½ grams of fat. You can use it instead of cinnamon in your favorite spice blend. Add a pinch or two to your tomato sauce for a flavor boost. Use it as a salt substitute in your sweet potatoes, bean soups and even in your eggs.

People with diabetes need to understand the power of intention. If things aren't working try something new. Develop new habits. This tip is good for everyone not just people with diabetes.

Party Survival Tips

1. Plan for the party ahead of time to prevent overeating. Try eating a small snack before going to the party.
2. Bring a healthy dish to the party so you will have something you can enjoy without worry.
3. Choose smaller serving at the party and stick to what you know you can eat!
4. Get up and get dancing and moving to the music. It burns calories and keeps you on track for another bite of something special.
5. Eat slowly remember it takes twenty minutes for the brain to get the message that you're full or satisfied.
6. Remember to eat smaller meals and stick to 4-5 hours apart before you eat.

Ways to Change ingredients in recipes to lower fat and sugar

It is possible to enjoy your favorite holiday fare without all of the calories, fat and sugar. Decrease the fat and sugar in recipes by 1/3 to ½ of the specified amount.

Use a sugar substitute in place of sugar in recipes. To enhance the sweet flavor use cinnamon, vanilla or nutmeg.

Substitute two egg whites or an egg substitute for each egg in recipes.

Use evaporated skim milk for cream.

Try reduced-fat margarine instead of butter when cooking.

Use unsweetened applesauce in place of some of the oil in baking goods.

Chill gravy or sauce, and then skim off the fat as it rises to the surface.

Season steam veggies with herbs or lemon juice in place of rich sauces. Use a fat free or reduced fat cream cheese or sour cream for mayonnaise.

I enjoy a glass of wine with my dinner or sometimes afterwards. But keep in mind that alcohol use needs to be monitored and that it is fattening if you drink too much!

Five ways to jazz up your water

1. Try flavored seltzer water. You can always buy plain and add your own fruit juices to flavor it up.
2. Add lemon or lime juice to your water.
3. Try individual serving size packets of sugar free flavored powder.
4. Add slices of fresh lemon, lime, orange, cucumber or watermelon to a glass of water.

5. Pour just a splash of fruit juice into seltzer water for a fruit juice spritzer.

Water and Seltzer
Water and seltzer water are your best choices because they contain nothing. No calories, no carbs and no fat. Your body need water to stay healthy.

Vegetable Juice
Not crazy about vegetables? You might like to try a vegetable juice or tomato juice. It low in calories and it's a great change of pace to a regular item.

Milk
Calcium has been found to help in reducing fat from the body. So drink milk or try using more calcium products in your regular diet.

Fruit Juice
Did you know that an eight ounce glass of orange juice has as many carbs as two small oranges? Be careful not to overdue the juice you don't want to put calories back on.

Sodas and Soft Drinks
It doesn't matter what soda or drink you choose they are all loaded with sodium; so be very careful try to stick to diet drinks but they are loaded with sodium too.

There is no order to the menus or recipes in this book. I did this so you would browse and look for things you haven't tried before. Here's a recipe for Pepper steak you will enjoy.

Legal Pepper Steak
1 tablespoon of olive oil
1 green pepper cut into strips
1 onion peeled and thinly sliced
1 pound of skirt or flank steak cut into strips
1 small bottle of chili sauce
¼ cup of water
2 tablespoons of Worcestershire sauce
¼ teaspoon salt substitute
¼ teaspoon of black pepper

In a large skillet heat oil over medium high heat. Add the pepper and onion; cook stirring often until it starts to brown. Transfer to a plate. Add the Beef to the skillet, cook stirring often until browned. Stir in the chili sauce, water, and Worcestershire; add peppers and onions and let simmer. Add the salt and pepper to taste. Try serving this steak with brown rice which has been cooked in a low sodium chicken broth.

Dehydration
Are you tired, cranky, headache or sluggish? Do you have dark urine or are you constipated? Drink more water the problem just might be that you are dehydrated.

Nausea and Vomiting
Did you eat or drink to fast? Over eat? Hard to digest your food? Try this simple trick…CHEW..CHEW… CHEW AND CHEW AGAIN. You just might be eating to fast so slow it down.

Having problems sticking to the diet? Maybe you need to remember that it takes time for the mind and the stomach to get in line with the program. Be patient it takes months for some people to get into a normal routine of eating. Remember to focus on eating protein at each meal this is great for our muscles, especially when it comes to toning and firming up later in the program.

Foods to Avoid
Whole milk
Full fat cheeses
Ice cream
Cheese Whiz
High fat processed meats
Beef brisket
Ribs
Fried meats
Bacon and sausage (only eat turkey products)
Prime rib
All margarine and butters
Crisco and vegetable oil
Full fat mayonnaise or Miracle Whip
All partially hydrogenated vegetable oils, trans fat
Regular soda and Kool-Aid (only unsweetened or sugar free)
Cookies, cakes and pastries (only sugar free is legal)
Barbeque sauces
White bread
Pasta (stick to whole wheat)
Bagels, doughnuts, Danish, croissants, pancakes
Saltine crackers
Fried vegetables

Sugar substitutes that are legal
Aspartame
Saccharin
Stevia
Sugar alcohols
Splenda

Drink a minimum of 64 ounces of non calorie and decaf fluids daily between meals every day! I know this seems like a lot but you need the water to flush the waste materials out of the body. The water will also help with hunger and will help keep you from overeating.

Want to know how to work food into your schedule try looking at this sample menu:

7am Breakfast
6 ounces of low sodium vegetable juice
¼ - ½ cup egg substitute (1 real egg)
2 slices of Canadian bacon
¼ cup mushrooms

10 am Snack
1 part skim-mozzarella cheese stick
5 whole wheat crackers

12:30 Lunch
Grilled chicken breast on romaine lettuce
¼ cup shredded low fat cheddar cheese
2 tablespoons Balsamic Vinaigrette
3 slices of tomatoes
½ cup cucumbers

3PM afternoon snack
Celery stuffed with 1 wedge of laughing cow cheese or 1
tablespoon peanut butter

5:30 Dinner
Grilled Salmon
Steamed asparagus
Tossed salad (spring greens, cucumbers, tomatoes,
green pepper)
2 Tablespoons low calorie dressing

8PM Snack
Low fat cottage cheese mixed with sugar free cherry
Jello and cool whip lithe topping

The time isn't important what is important is the way
you incorporate food into your daily diet! You need to try
increasing your protein to 60-80 grams per day. This is
very important when it comes to the toning of the muscles
later. I know I do a lot of repeating but there are some
things which are very important if you want to succeed
and reach your goal weight. Even more important is the
fact I want you to keep in mind that as the weight comes
off you will have to make adjustments in your life. You
may find that you for instance had big boobs all your life,
but after losing the weight your boobs shrunk. I found this
to be disturbing and even though I always had too much
backside, I lost my entire backside and I just didn't know
how to react to all of it. I hadn't planned on my emotions
getting involved; I thought I was going to love everything
about my weight loss but the truth of the matter is I
didn't and I found it to be disturbing to look at. If you

can afford the surgery to get the boob job then you're lucky; I couldn't so my breasts have to be rebuilt up with weight training. I hope that you will consider this when dieting and if you find you don't exactly like how you are looking; then stop and readjust your thinking. The weight off is better than the weight on and if looks were all you were trying to do this for then prepare yourself for a total shock. How we look is not going to change the inside of the mind so remember to exercise and to keep smiling. After all a small backside is better than one sticking out a mile long! Beauty is in the eye of the beholder, though this statement leaves room for change it does sum things up rather tightly. How you accept your new body and the changes that comes with it becomes the most important part of dieting. If you have only a few pounds to lose this probably won't affect you, but if you were like me and have a great deal of weight to lose; you need to start now accepting that everything is not going to be a bed of roses. My personal relationship changed because my friend who was never jealous became very jealous and that was more depressing than not having the big backside! You have to work at accepting yourself and it takes time I still have problems after three years with accepting my new look. I hope that you will seek professional help if you see that it is too hard for you to adjust to. You are not going to put the weight back on you are going to learn to live with the changes. With weight loss comes and mental change and adjustment and if you can't accept the change you will find yourself gaining the weight back. I met a lady who went through the painful surgery and lost weight and reached her goal weight; only her family teased her so hard that she started gaining the weight back. She now is over fifty pounds overweight again and had to start all over again losing. Only this time she is learning to eat the weight off and learning portion control. She told me that she had been so use to having someone do it for herself that she didn't realize she didn't know how to achieve her goal without surgery. You can only have the surgery once so she had to resort to learning what she should have learned in the first place. She told me that if she had taken the time to learn weight control properly and learn how to fix the food for her she wouldn't have gained the weight back. She's right it's easy to maintain when you know what you are doing and how it's done. Not everything is good for you as they claim especially if your finances run out like hers did.

Calories always count. Looking at labels and being familiar with label terminology will enhance your weight loss experience. Please keep in mind that calories and portion sizes still count. Sugar free does not mean calorie free!

I'm no expert but here are some cooking tips which helped me along my journey:

Recipe calls for	Replace it with
Two eggs	three eggs whites
One cup of Cheddar cheese	one cup of fat free Cheddar shredded
One cup of whole milk	cup skim milk
One cup of mayonnaise	one cup of fat free Mayonnaise
One cup of cream	cup of evaporated Skim milk
Cup of sour cream	cup of fat free cream Or a cup of cottage Cheese blended with Lemon juice

Healthy Cooking Tips

Poaching
Poaching uses a shallow pan of boiling water to quickly cook foods such as eggs and fish. Your food will be moist, tender, and have no added fat.

Steaming
Steaming is an excellent way to cook most vegetables, and even some fruits. There are two ways to steam. The old fashion way is to use a pot or pan where you place your food in a small amount of boiling water to create steam that cooks the food. With the recommended vegetables, plan to fully steam them to make the food easier to chew and digest.

Another way to steam is to place your food in a microwavable plate or bowl, cover it with plastic wrap, and microwave it. The microwave will use the moisture already in the food to steam the food.

Boiling

Boiling is easy, requires little attention, and is great for meats and vegetables. It's an excellent way to cook anything to make it soft enough to mash or put in a blender.

Baking or Roasting

Oven baking is a great alternative to frying. If possible use a rack to raise your food above the bottom of the pan to keep it out of the fat drippings. Can use the dollar store racks inside of the pan they work perfect and the food is moist.

Stir-Frying

There is a low calorie way to stir fry by either using a non stick pan or wok, or using a small amount of olive oil or spray oil. Remember to cook on a medium high or high heat and allow the food to cook effectively.

Grilling and Broiling

You can grill or broil meat or vegetables on an indoor grill or backyard grill. Make sure the meat is well trimmed of fat, and for poultry the skin is removed. Grill slowly so that the meat doesn't dry out.

It took three years and half for me to lose the weight and I still am trying to firm up the loose skin. I want you to understand that even after you reaching your goal weight there will still be more work for you to do. I can't afford the surgery needed to get rid of all of the loose skin so I have to work at toning it. You will notice I said I have to still work at toning and you will more than likely have to do the same. I have been toning my body for over a year and though I have made some progress I still have a long way to go. You can't get upset just because you lose the weight and your body isn't perfect. I want you to realize that there is still a process after the weight is gone. I am not sure if I can tone away all the excess skin but I am attempting to do just that. As you head towards your goal I will right be there hoping you don't become disillusion and that you will stay focus on reaching your goal. The journey is really just beginning and you have everything to reach for. This weight is only the first step in a series of many. Good luck and don't give up until you too reach your goal weight. For more information or more recipes and tips feel free to contact Wilfred's web page or e-mail us at anytime. Good Luck and good eating. "Remember we're getting healthier one step at a time."

WALKFREE is a license rotating health club which can be reached through e-mail. Write me and let me know how you are doing I look forward to hearing from you. Once again losing the weight is just the beginning of a journey yet to come. Nothing is impossible after all I lost 370 pounds and you too can reach your goal with time. Don't give up...stay focus and you too will reach your goal no matter whether it is one pound or five hundred. The joy is in reaching your goal and that is a reality that the future holds. Remember that you have to stick to monitoring your intake of food but don't let it consume you. Healthy eating is only the first step to succeeding. Once again I say GOOD LUCK AND GOOD EATING.

You can e-mail me Walkfreehealthclub@msn/live.com Or if you want to know more about WALKFREE ROTATING HEALTH CLUB, look us at www.walkfreerotatinghealthclub.com I look forward to hearing how you are doing. Need a new recipe or tips, I will e-mail you one back. This journey is one that you are not alone on so don't give up!

The book What Weight was designed to help you along with your diet. The book was designed to motivate you into learning more about how to lose weight and how to keep yourself at your goal weight. J. M. Clark has been doing motivational talking and showing individuals how to lose weight and more important how to eat the weight off. She talks about personal problems she encountered along the way, during her weight lost. The goal of the book is to encourage you not to stop trying because you face a minor failure or set back. You will find recipes designed to help you stay on track. The food is designed on a 300 calorie or less meal. It is designed to help you see that just about any food can be cut down or changed to lesser calories. You will find that when problems come up you will now have a short guideline as to what to do so you can get back on track. There is no right or wrong to this diet plan mainly because it is a book designed to help you along with your diet program. You are encouraged to show the program to your diet specialist or doctor for his approval as a self help book. Remember that you have to use the book along with your diet program, it is not designed to be used along but has and you can do just that. Motivation is important in losing weight and understanding that even the best dieter's have moments where they need a little push. It is important to understand when you have an embarrassing moment that everyone does and that it is then you should right away focus on getting back on track. Turn those embarrassing moments into moments of success and focus on making the next moment a successful one. Remember you can succeed all it takes is a few moments of resetting your mind. What you think is important when it comes to making right choices. I hope this book will be a help mate to you and that you will find it to be a great referral book on your road to success in losing. Good Luck.